Thank You For Buying This Book
'CHANGES'
PUBERTY, ONLINE EDUCATION FOR YOUR CHILD AND FAMILY

This book has a support Three Session Series CD or link via email download which will be sent to you.

Please contact, admin@fullpotentialtraining.com.au with your email contact information and we will send you all necessary information.

If we are sending the course via CD, we will need your complete home physical address. Please see the attached form, please fill in and return to the above email address.

Thank you again, Christine.

Our Mission:
Every child and adult have value and is important to us; therefore, we strive through research, online education, and book publishing, to bring life-skill education to all children and all families.

For Education Packages

Please see our book website:
www.how2books.com.au and
Education packages,
www.fullpotentialtraining.com.au
or Contact:
admin@fullpotentialtraining.com.au

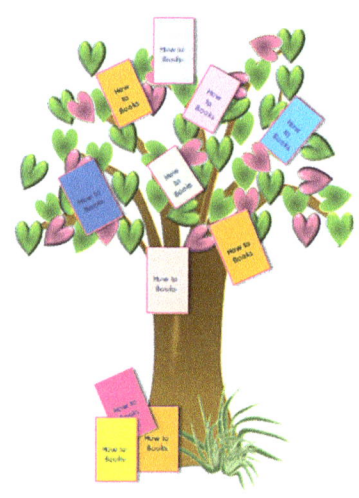

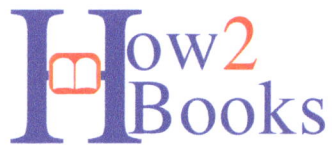

If you have purchased this book without its cover, it may be a stolen book.

Neither the publisher or the author is under any obligation to provide professional services in anyway, legal, health or in any form which is related to this book, its contents advice or otherwise.

The law and practices vary from country to country and state to state.

If legal or professional information is required, the purchaser, or the reader should seek the information privately and best suited to their particular needs, and circumstances.

This is not a medical book. It is a book developed by the publisher to open the conversation about how the human body changes when growing up.

The author and publisher specifically disclaim any liability that may be incurred from the information within this book.
All rights reserved. No part of this book, including the interior design, images, cover design, diagrams, or any intellectual property (IP), icons and photographs may be reproduced or transmitted in any form by any means (electronic, photocopying, recording or otherwise) without the prior permission of the publisher. ©

Copyright© 2022 MSI Australia
All rights reserved.
ISBN: 978-0-6457284-1-5

Published by How2Books
Under licence from MSI Ltd, Australia
Company Registration No: 96963518255
NSW, Australia
See our website: www.how2books.com.au
Or contact by email: sales@how2books.com.au
Covers and Copyright owned by MSI, Australia

MSI acknowledges the author and images, text and photographs used in this book.

WORKBOOK

ONLINE PUBERTY EDUCATION

11 14 & up to 18 YEARS

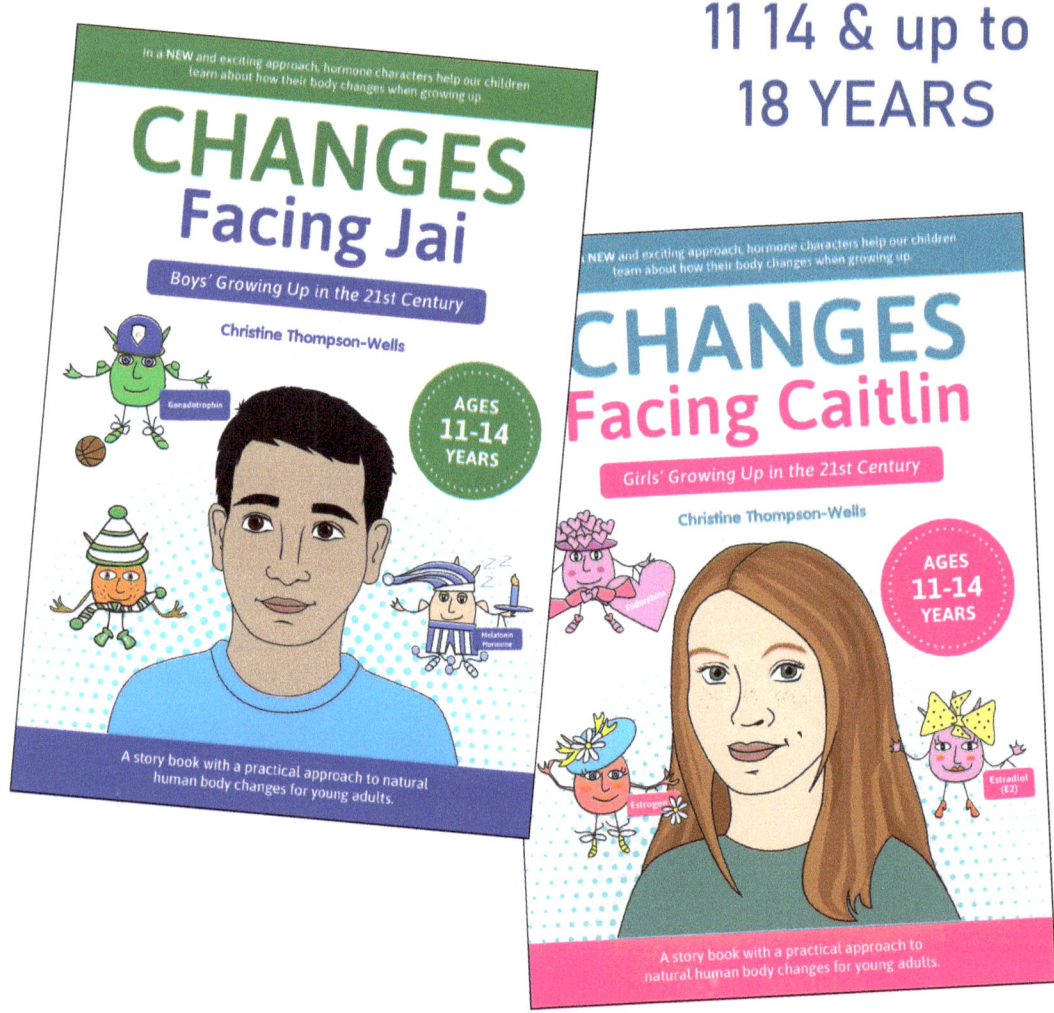

HOME LEARNING FOR YOU AND YOUR FAMILY
....
YOUR NAME
....

SESSION ONE

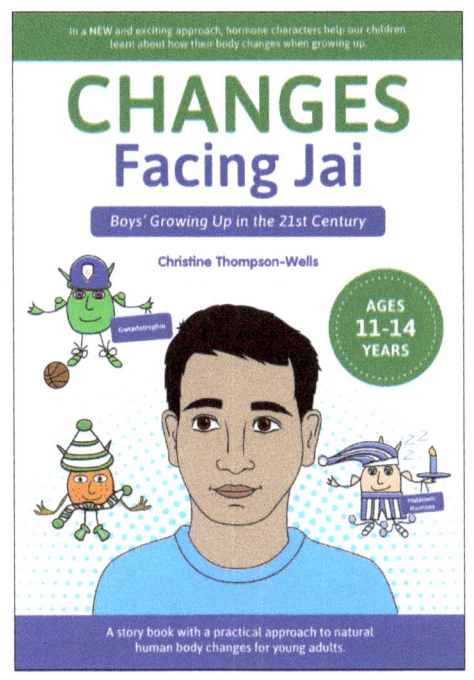 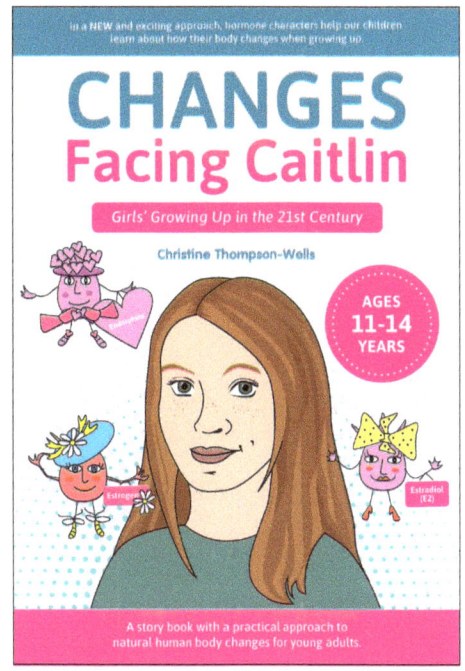

HORMONES WITH HATS – IT'S ALL ABOUT HORMOMES

SLIDE ONE – WELCOME – ONLINE PUBERTY EDUCATION

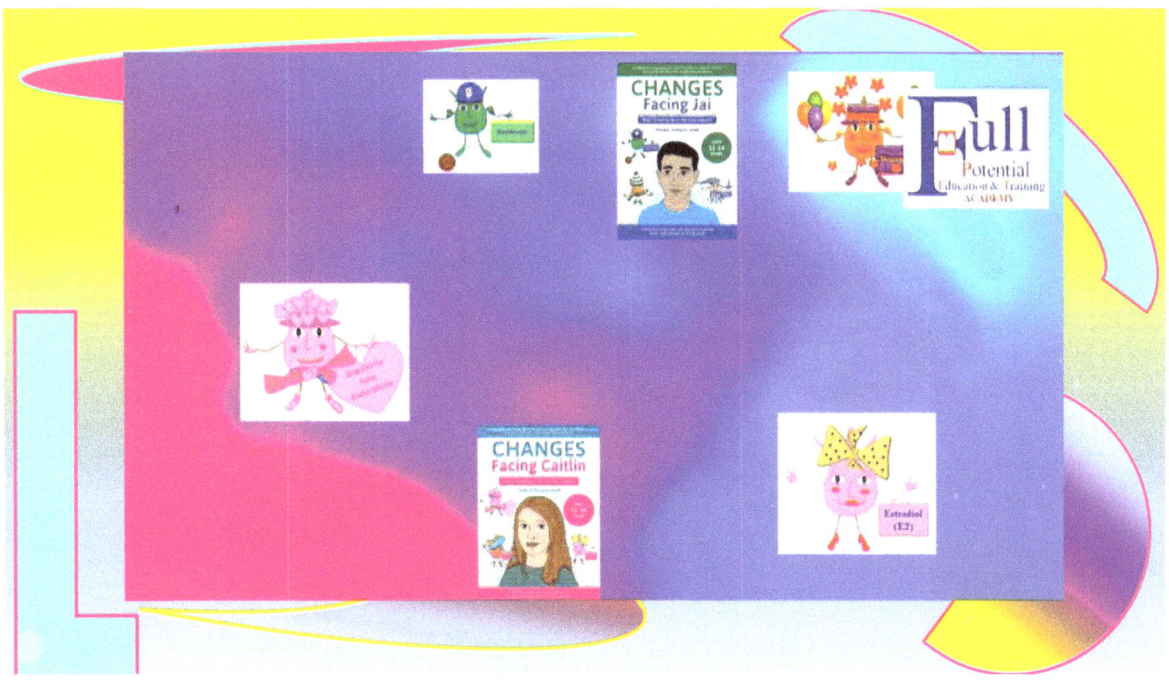

SLIDE TWO – INTRODUCTION VIDEO

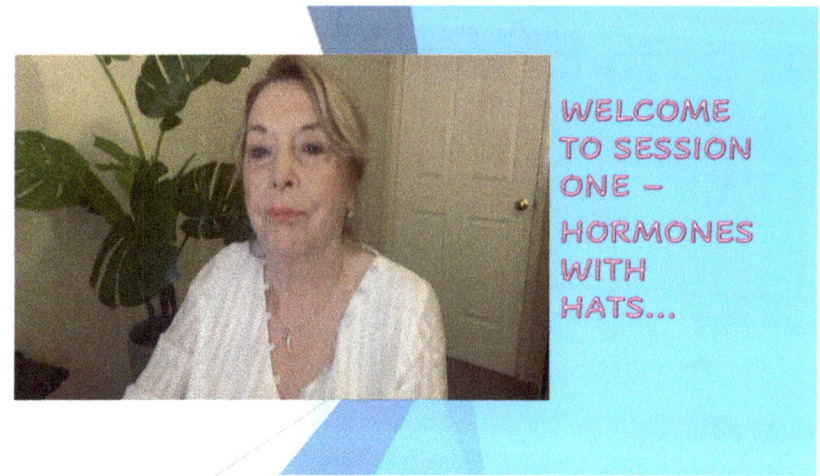

SLIDE THREE – THE OBJECTIVES AND OUTCOMES FOR THE SESSION

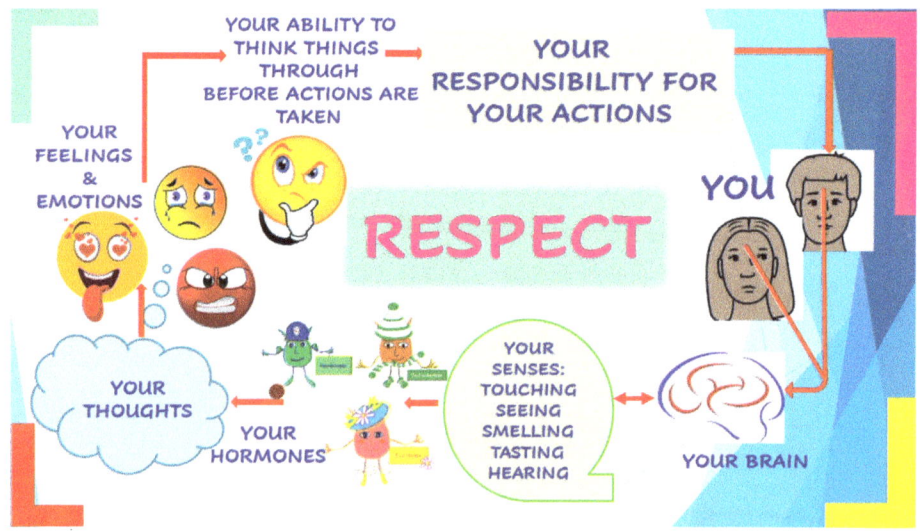

SLIDE FOUR – THE CYCLE OF YOU

Taking a minute to understand the route of the journey.

Understanding how your body works will help to keep you safe, while growing up. With this knowledge, you become aware of the stages the body takes, from growing to a child, young adult, then to mature adult.

SLIDE FIVE - THE GROWTH HORMONE

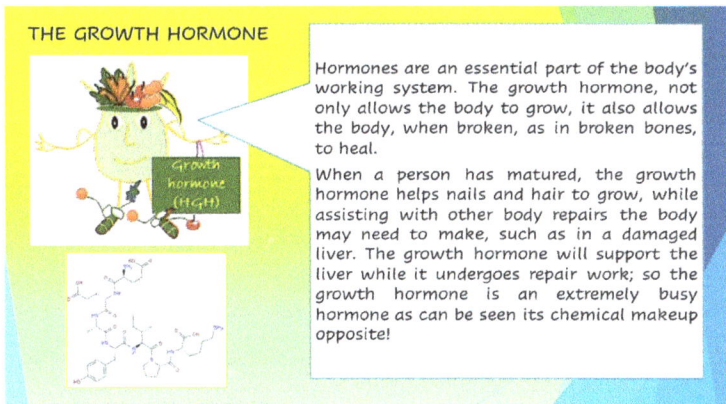

Many hormones give support to other working hormones in your body… The human body is an intricate system of many working systems. Each system works with the other systems in your body. If you can imagine, the London underground in the United Kingdom, the trains run, usually, on time without accident! If one train has a breakdown, many trains on different lines become disrupted. Your body's system is far more complicated than that, therefore, when one part of your system/s is disrupted, other parts may breakdown…! Drugs, alcohol, junk food and other negative habits, can all interfere with your body's system!

Science, with hard core evidence, is giving us information about many young people suffering with their body's systems because of poor eating, and soft drink habits. This includes interfering with the growth hormone…!

YOUR NOTES
....
....
....

SLIDE SIX – TESTOSTERONE HORMONE

In females, testosterone is produced in the ovaries and adrenal glands. In males, it is also produced in the testes and adrenal glands and is key to a healthy prostate gland. In both males and females, testosterone is an important hormone in

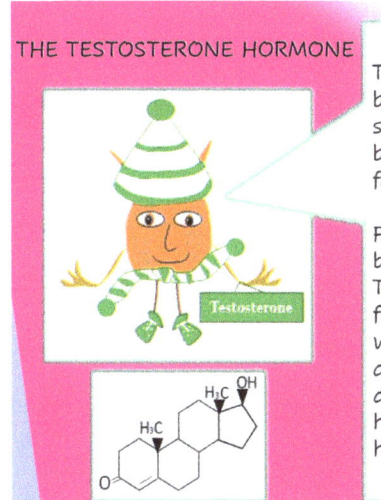

both brain and heart health.

In males, it plays a key role in reproduction. Low levels of testosterone have been attributed to food additives, including colouring dyes and other processed foods and drinks.

YOUR NOTES

....
....
....
....
....
....
....
....
....
....

SLIDE SEVEN – GONADOTROPIN HORMONE

The hormone Gonadotropin's main function is to help to control the functions within the ovaries and testes.

Gonadotropins are important for the regulation and proper functioning related to male and female reproduction.

The main function of gonadotropins is to work with the gonads, meaning, the gonad is the sex reproductive gland in both males and females.

Gonadotropins are made in the pituitary gland in response to other hormone stimulation in the hypothalamus in your brain. The process of production is carried out by the hypothalamus pituitary gonad axis.

YOUR NOTES

....
....
....
....
....

SLIDE EIGHT – LOOKING AT HOW IT WORKS!

The Gonads are a part of the endocrine system, they are known as the male and female reproductive hormones.

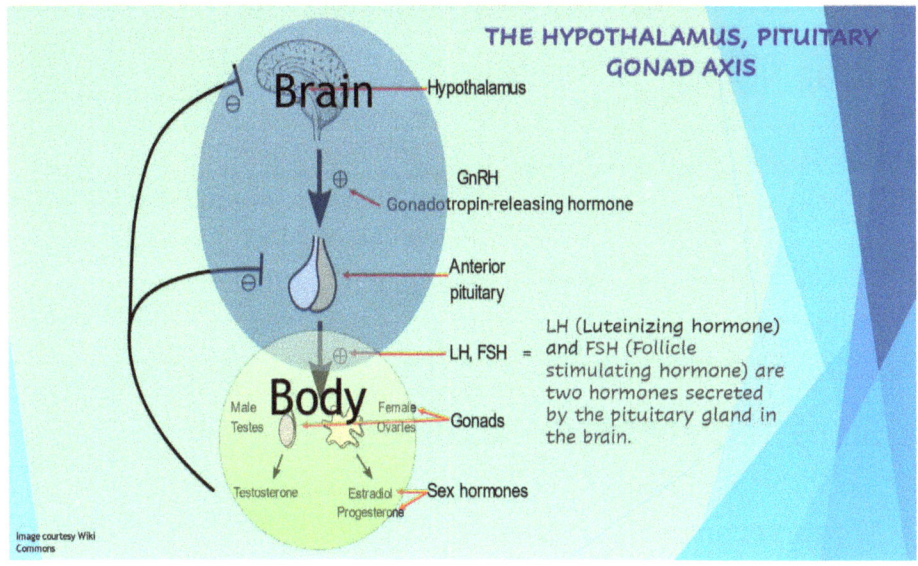

Ovaries are the female gonad while testes are the male gonad; they are responsible for producing sex hormones in our bodies.

YOUR NOTES

....
....
....
....
....
....
....

SLIDE NINE – ESTROGEN HORMONE

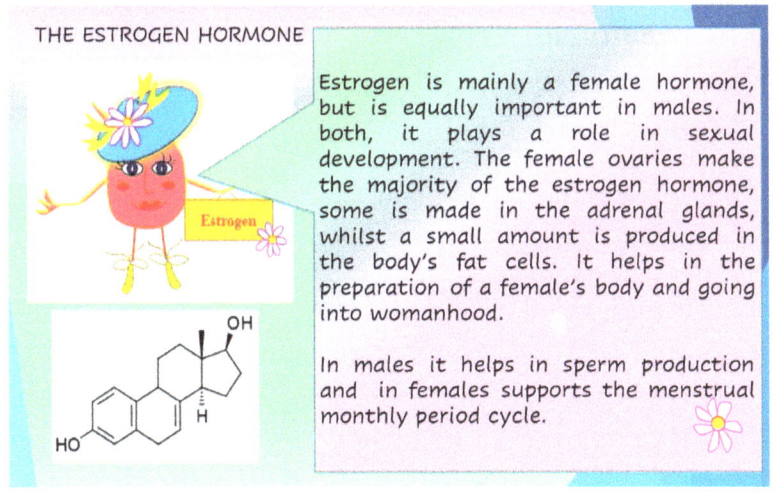

Estrogen is needed in both the female and male body systems. It not only supports the body the grow and change in puberty, but contributes to blood vessel support, brain and skin health, female breast development and pelvic muscle support.

It is, in part, supportive of hair growth in the pubic and armpit areas of males and females. It contributes to the wellbeing of your cardiovascular and bone development.

Some foods that support the estrogen hormone, include alfalfa sprouts, flax seeds, fennel, sesame seeds, garlic, peaches, wheat bran, whole grain breads, fresh berries, naturally dried fruits, and soybeans.

YOUR NOTES

....
....
....
....
....
....
....

SLIDE TEN - PROGESTERONE HORMONE

Progesterone is released from the female ovaries. It helps when females start to have their periods, and in the body's control of the menstrual cycle. It is released from the female ovaries. It helps when females start to have their periods, and in the body's control of the menstrual cycle. In males, it is the precursor to testosterone production, it also helps to balance male estrogen.

In males, the balance between testosterone, progesterone and male estrogen is the key to being a healthy male.

YOUR NOTES

....
....
....
....
....
....
....
....
....
....
....

SLIDE ELEVEN - ESTRONE HORMONE

Estrone can store estrogen and helps with female development and plays a part in female reproductive health. Like most hormones, these work with the body's clock.

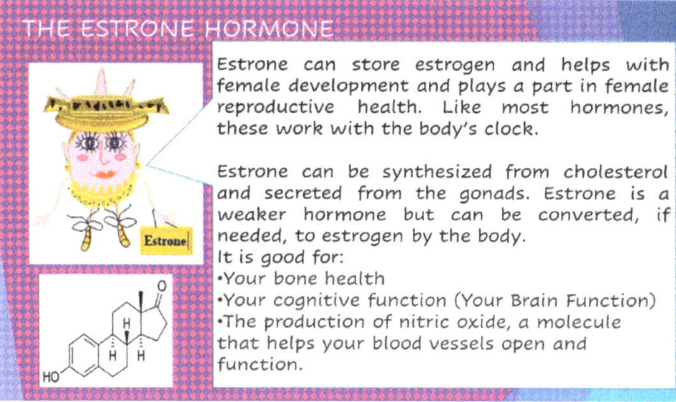

Estrone can be synthesized from cholesterol and secreted from the gonads and from the body's fatty tissue. Estrone is a weaker hormone than estrogen but can be converted, if needed, to estrogen by the body.

It is good for:
- Your bone health
- Cognitive function (Your Brain Function) &
- The production of nitric oxide, a molecule that helps blood vessels open and function.

YOUR NOTES
....
....

All the hormones in your body and brain need to work in balance; many hormones work with more than one hormone for effective body functions.

Each hormone needs to be positively fuelled by the food you eat. Your body, though you are living in the 21st Century, is an ancient system that has taken many thousands of years of evolution to make it what it is today.

Your body responds positively to whole food, not processed, artificial food made from many synthetic ingredients!

SLIDE TWELVE – ESTRIOL HORMONE

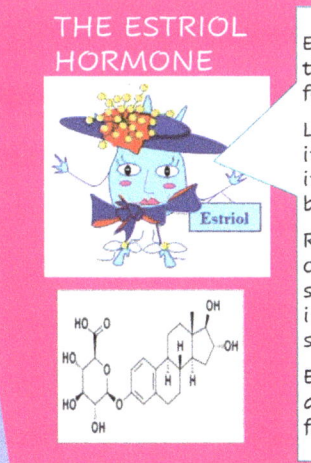

Estriol, like estrone, and estradiol, helps the female body to grow and become ready for womanhood.

Like so many hormones, it too,

works with its own clock and will click into gear when it receives certain messages from your brain. Quantities of this hormone are high in females during pregnancy with its highest levels being before and during childbirth.

Research is revealing, Estriol appears to offer a wide range of health benefits to several health conditions, some of which include rheumatoid arthritis, multiple sclerosis, thyroiditis, and psoriasis.

In men, it is found in the fatty tissue of the testicles, and in their fatty brain tissue.

YOUR NOTES

....
....
....
....
....

SLIDE THIRTEEN – ESTRADIOL HORMONE

Estradiol is principally a female hormone, produced primarily in the female ovaries.

Estradiol levels can vary depending on the phase of the female menstrual cycle.

It is also involved with the adjustment of the female reproductive cycles.

It helps the female body in the maintenance of the reproductive tissue within the uterus and the breasts.

Estradiol helps maintain memory, increases sexual interest in males and females, improves mood and happiness and improves sleep quality.

In Males, it regulates sex drive, helps in achieving erections, the production of sperm and testicular function.

YOUR NOTES

....
....
....

SLIDE FOURTEEN – GHRELIN HORMONE

Ghrelin is the hormone that lets you know when you feel hungry. If people eat when they are not hungry, for instance, junk food can make you feel full and about an hour later after the meal, you feel hungry again! When this happens, your ghrelin hormone release may become confused.

Your gut sends a message to your brain saying, 'I'm hungry.' The message is received by the hypothalamus in the brain. The hypothalamus helps in the regulation of many hormones, and ghrelin is just one!

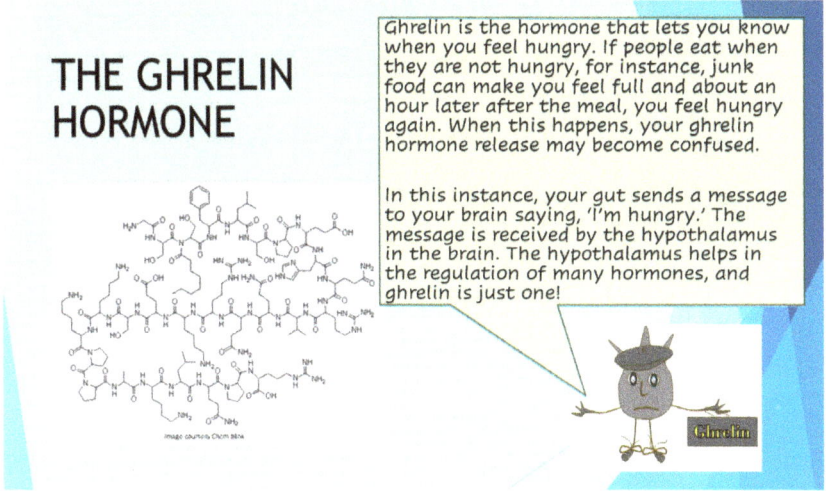

Ghrelin's main function is to increase appetite and encourages eating more food than is possibly necessary for a healthy body to function. The nature of the hormone may encourage eating more calorie foods which are stored in the body's fat, thus increasing weight if the extra calories are not used in work or exercise!

During puberty, the body and brain are changing and can grow exponentially! This growth puts extra demands on the body and for you to eat more food than is possibly needed! The instant feelings of satisfaction given by junk food will encourage you to eat non-healthy food because of the instant rewards of satisfaction given to your brain!

YOUR NOTES

....
....
....
....
....
....
....
....
....
....
....
....

SLIDE FIFTEEN – GHRELIN HORMONE CONTINUED

The higher levels of ghrelin, the hungrier you become! Woven into the demands of this hormone's work, maybe the eating habits of junk or processed food.

....
....
....
....
....
....
....

YOUR NOTES

....
....
....

SLIDE SIXTEEN – GETTING TO KNOW ADRENALINE

The adrenal hormone gland is responsible for making many hormones, including, cortisol, aldosterone, adrenaline, and noradrenaline. The adrenaline gland is controlled by the pituitary gland in the brain.

As you may be aware, adrenaline is also known as the 'fight or flight' hormone, though helpful in times of stress, too much adrenalin can make you anxious, nervous, or excited, therefore, it is important to manage adrenalin and like hormones.

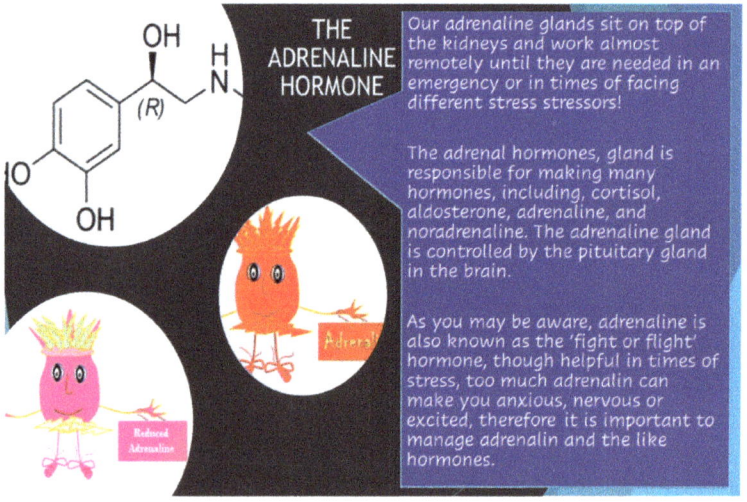

When you feel you are under attack, either physically or emotionally, your adrenaline level will rise, some signs to look for: nervous tension or irritability, dilated pupils, rapid heart rate and breathing, sweating in the palm of your hands or feet, a heightened senses showing reluctance to go to school, college, or university.

A way of managing too much adrenalin is through sport, exercise, meditation or breathing exercises.

YOUR NOTES
....
....
....

SLIDE SEVENTEEN – GETTING TO KNOW CORTISOL

Cortisol is sometimes referred to as the stress hormone; it is naturally occurring and made by the adrenal gland. The hormone is used throughout the body which is controlled by the hypothalamus.

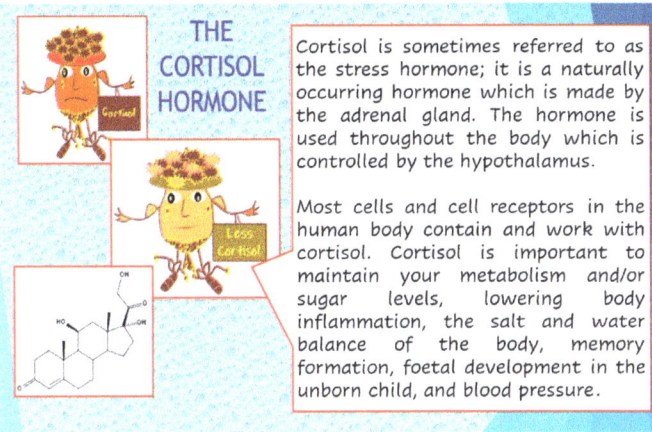

Most cells and cell receptors in the human body contain and work with cortisol.

Cortisol is important to maintain your metabolism and/or sugar levels, lowering body inflammation, the salt and water balance of the body, memory formation, foetal development in the unborn child, and blood pressure.

YOUR NOTES
....
....
....

SLIDE EIGHTEEN – GETTING TO KNOW SEROTONIN

Serotonin is known as the 'Happiness' hormone. It helps with mood adjustment, developing regular sleep patterns, bone health, helps wounds or cut skin to heal, supports your digestive system, helps with learning and academic attainment; it

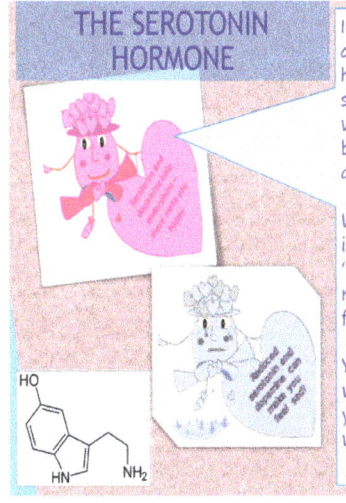

also helps with libido, or sexual drive, and desire.

YOUR NOTES
....
....
....

Now, please do the following exercise.

Your Feeling And Emotional Gauge

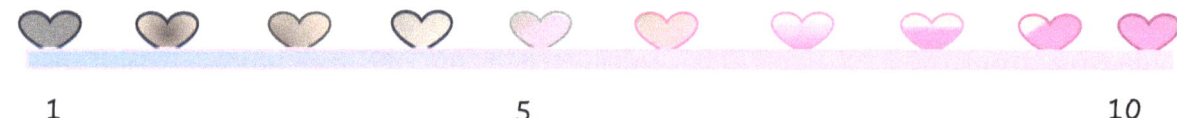

SLIDE NINETEEN - **YOUR FEELING AND EMOTIONAL GAUGE**

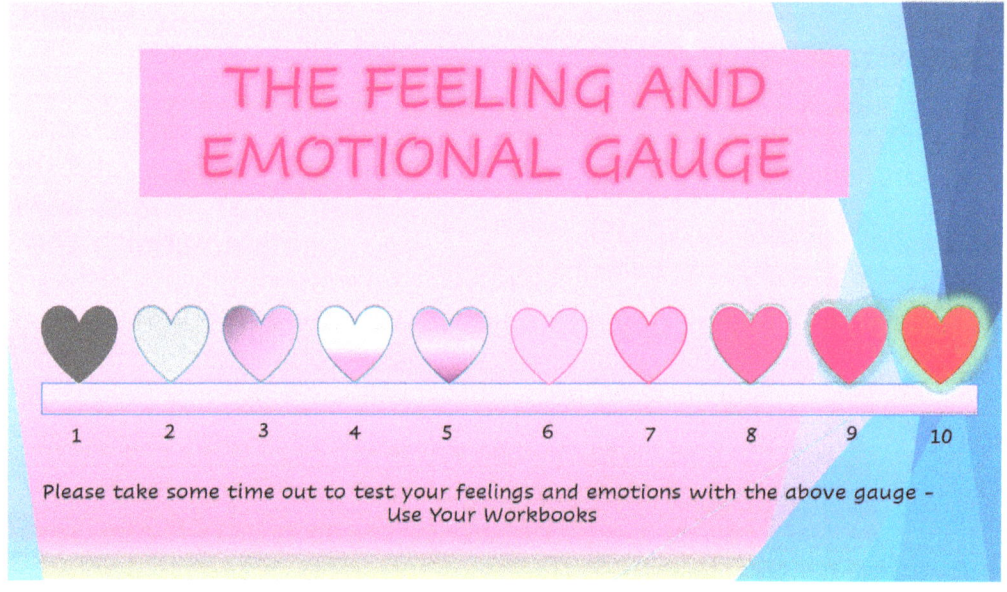

1) Not a good place, take some time out, do some sport or physical activity like walking or swimming.

5) You are feeling better but could go backwards unless you keep yourself occupied and busy. Always have a project or sport you can work on; this will keep your mind active.

6) You are managing everyday life demands and are confident in your capabilities.

10) You are in love; you may be infatuated and all you think about is another person. Try to come down to 7 or 8 on the Feeling and Emotional Gauge. Infatuation is an emotion that can overcrowd your

feelings; you may lose your concentration *on schoolwork and other* life demands. This time will pass as your brain and body develop.

If you can, this is a good opportunity to have a family or discussion with a friend.

Balanced serotonin levels help with mood adjustment, developing regular sleep patterns, bone health, helps wounds or cut skin to heal, supports your digestive system, helps with learning and academic attainment, but it too, helps with libido, or sexual drive, and desire.

When serotonin is balanced and working in the human body, it also helps with 'happiness' feelings. When serotonin is not balanced, you will know by the feelings of sadness.

You can monitor your serotonin levels to measure how you feel...

If you measure between 1-4 on the gauge, please speak to a professional advisor, or somebody you trust.

YOUR NOTES
....
....
....
....

SLIDE TWENTY – GETTING TO KNOW OXYTOCIN

If a male or female has unrequited love, and if the feelings are not managed, this can lead to other emotional states and the body's reaction, which include, stress, poor self-esteem, lack of sleeping properly, isolation and lack of confidence. Other outcomes of this include limited touching, and 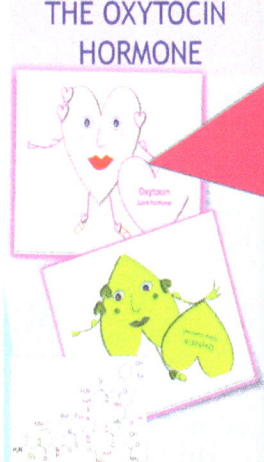 feelings of abandonment. Remedies for this situation include,

- ✓ go out with other people, you don't have to be in love with a person to enjoy their company.
- ✓ hobbies and projects are great to have when life seems like hell on the other side of the front door!

✓ reconnect with old friends, and importantly, reconnect with family members.

DO NOT TAKE REVENGE IF YOU ARE HURT, BE CREATIVE AND FIND ANOTHER DIRECTION

YOUR NOTES

....
....
....
....

SLIDE TWENTY-ONE – GETTING TO KNOW DOPAMINE – THE PARTY HORMONE

When there are high levels of dopamine in the brain, you will want to 'party!'

Continuous partying is not good for your health, brain, or study time. When dopamine becomes 'overcharged' – this happens in drug, alcohol, vaping or through other abuse substances, the brain creates a habit to 'party…!'

However, when dopamine is balanced, it helps with the following: focus and attention to different jobs, develop skills such as driving a car, and operating machinery, it helps you to study for examinations, and contributes to your motivation, to good mood and sleep patterns.

Dopamine assists with control of nausea or vomiting and how we process pain. It assists with blood vessel and kidney function and movement and assists with your heart rate. It also assists with memory function and how long information will stay in either the short or long-term memory.

YOUR NOTES

....
....
....
....
....

TWENTY-TWO – GETTING TO KNOW MELATONIN – THE SLEEP HORMONE

Melatonin is made in the pineal gland, a small pea-sized gland, found in the middle of the human mid-brain in the brain.

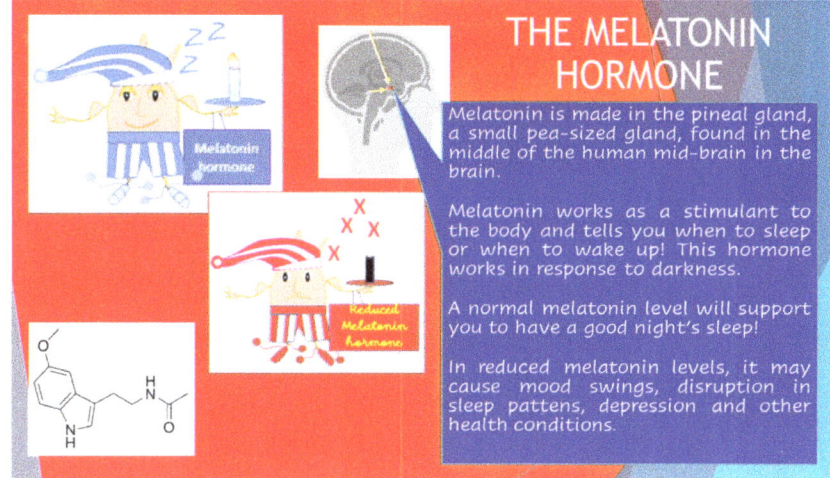

Melatonin works as a stimulant to the body and tells you when to sleep or when to wake up!

This hormone works in response to darkness. A normal melatonin level will support you to have a good night's sleep! In reduced melatonin levels, it may cause mood swings, disruption in sleep pattens, depression and other health conditions.

YOUR NOTES
....
....
....
....
....

SLIDE TWENTY-THREE – DISCUSSION – LET'S TALK
....
....
....

QUESTIONS TO BE ASKED

WHY ARE HORMONES IMPORTANT IN THE HUMAN BODY?
....
....
....

WHAT ROLE DOES TESTOSTERONE PLAY IN THE MALE BODY?
....
....
....
....
....
....

WHY IS ESTROGEN IMPORTANT TO THE FEMALE BODY?
....
....
....

WHY IS IT IMPORTANT TO UNDERSTAND THE INFORMATION ABOUT GHRELIN?
....
....
....

WHAT IS THE DIFFERENCE TO THE BODY WHEN EATING JUNK FOOD COMPARED TO EATING WHOLE FOOD?
....
....
....

SLIDE TWENTY-THREE -PLENARY

PLENARY & REFLECTION ON THE INFORMATION YOU HAVE LEARNT

- ✓ Hormones are chemical messengers that work within your body and brain!
- ✓ Eating 'junk food & drink can interfere with how your Hormones naturally work!
- ✓ Exercise can help to keep your hormones healthy & contribute to your positive wellbeing!
- ✓ Hormones are not only messengers, they are chemical compounds that respond to your senses and will let you know when you are in danger!
- ✓ Now, please add this information to your notes and
- ✓ Discuss with your class or group!

YOUR NOTES
....
....
....
....
....
....
....
....
....
....

END OF SESSION ONE

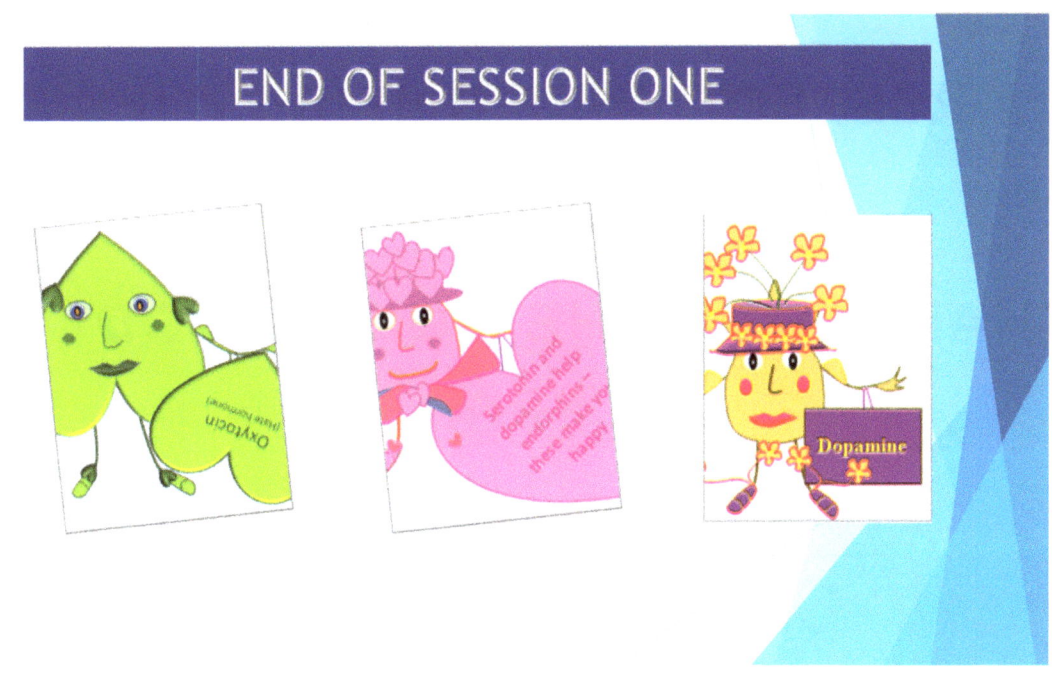

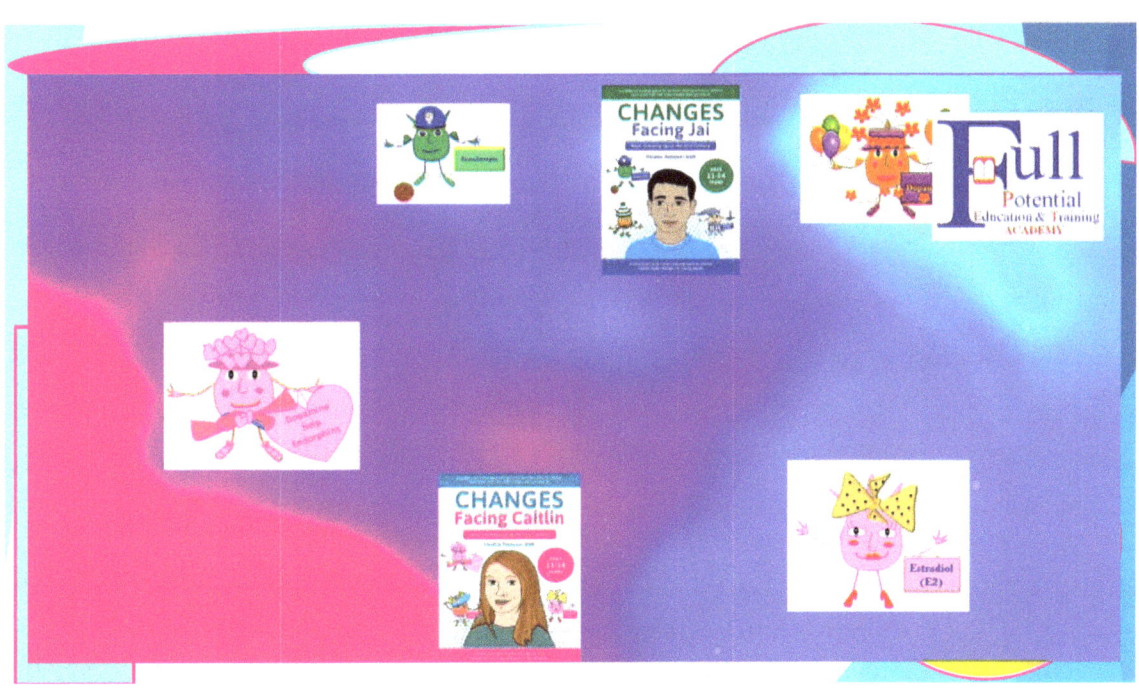

SESSION TWO

RESPECT, RESPONSIBILITIES & HORMONES

CHANGES TO THE HUMAN BODY AND BRAIN

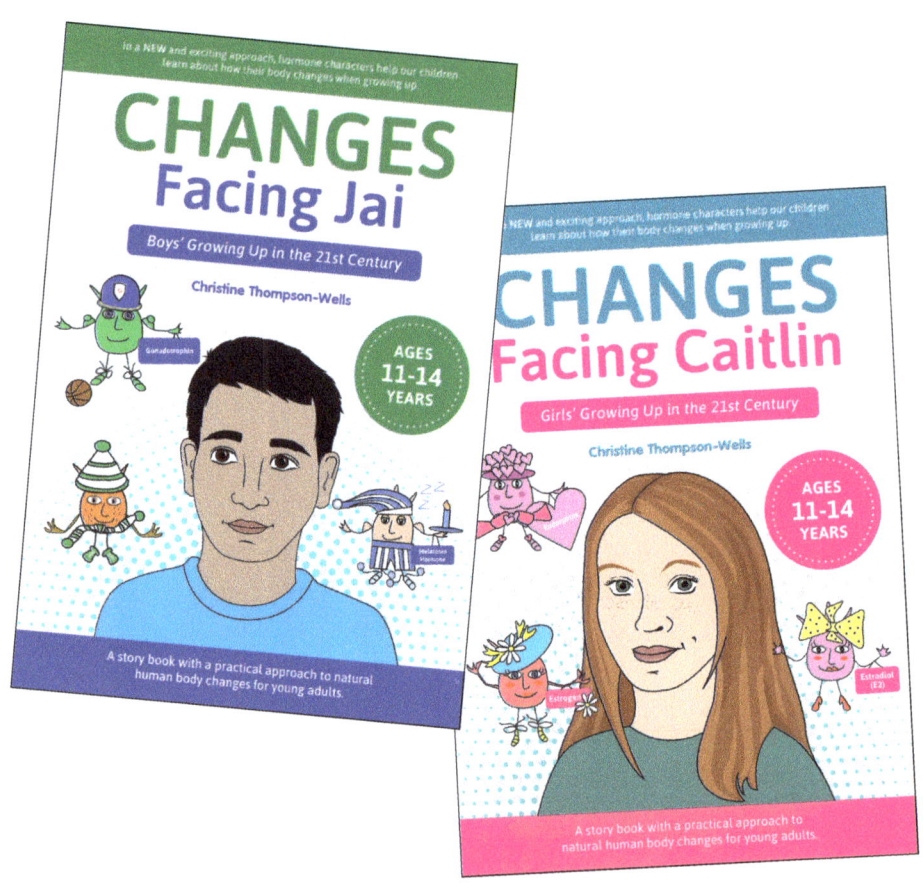

LET'S GET STARTED...!

WELCOME
SLIDE ONE – SESSION TWO

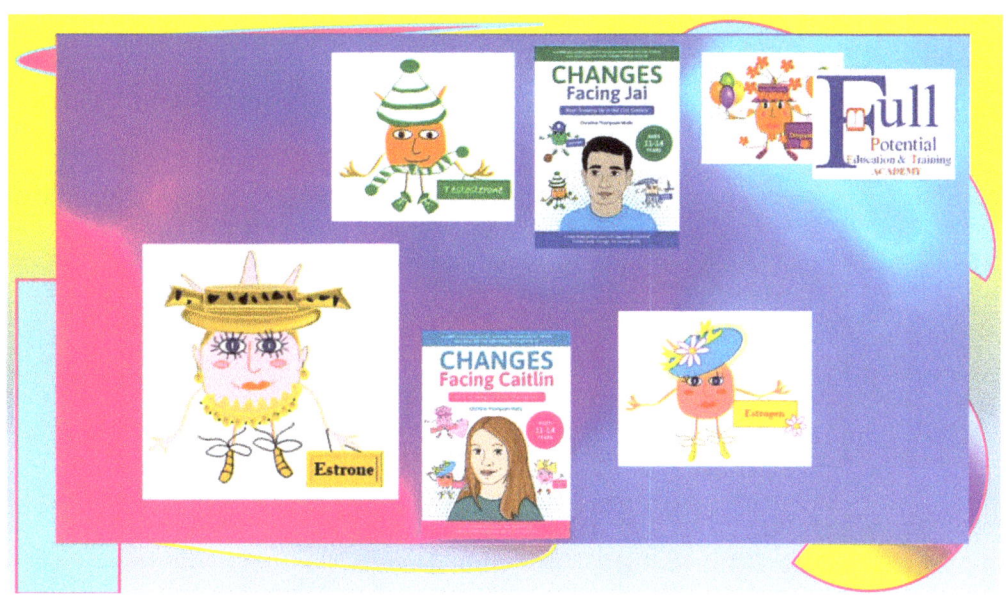

SLIDE TWO – INTRODUCTION

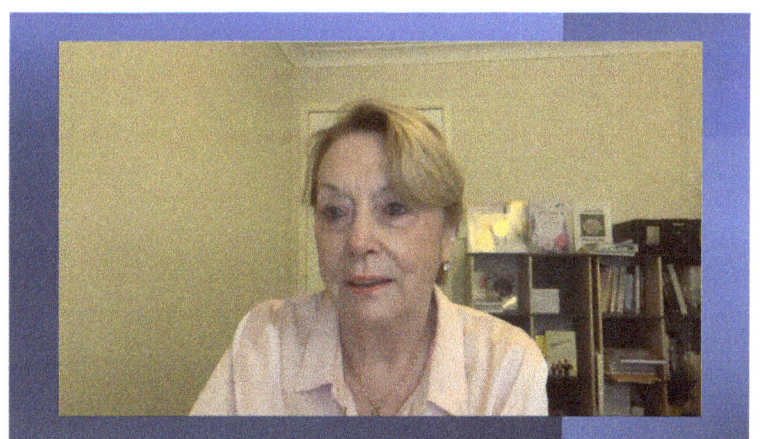

SLIDE THREE – SESSION TWO – OBJECTIVES AND OUTCOMES

SESSION TWO

RESPECT, RESPONSIBILITIES, HORMONES CHANGES TO THE HUMAN BODY AND BRAIN

THE OBJECTIVES AND OUTCOME FOR THE SESSION

By the end of the session, you the student, will have an understanding of how your brain and thinking go through different stages as you leave your childhood and head into adulthood. You will start to understand the meaning of the 'Dual Systems' of thinking and behaving.

You will become familiar with the correct terminology for different parts of your body and start to understand the complexity of these parts.

Remembering respect, we will identify both the female and male bodies and how they function.

Puberty is all about becoming aware of your body and brain changes, and the responsibilities that come into your life as you start to grow and change.

YOUR NOTES

....
....
....

SLIDE FOUR – RESPECT, RESPONSIBILITIES & HORMONES, CHANGES TO THE HUMAN BODY AND BRAIN

Not all hormones are designed to work in your body every day and every night, some work on specific timeclocks that are regulated by your age and life experiences. Puberty is regulated by your age timeline and is possibly handed down from your ancestors.

Many characteristics seen in children are seen in older adults such as grandparents. Some children have similar traits in actions, facial expressions, or mannerisms often seen in the older generations. Please take a moment, with your group to discuss an instance where your parents, aunt, uncle, or grandparents have said, 'You are just like…………………………. –

DISCUSSION...
....
....
....
....
....

SLIDE FIVE – WHAT IS THE MEANING OF RESPECT?

Respect has a great deal of meaning, some of which are:

1) Recognition of that person,
2) Value of that person,
3) Regard for that person,

4) Value of that person,
5) Pay attention to that person, and when they say 'NO', they mean 'NO'.
6) You will protect that person if you need to,
7) Show consideration for that person.

There are many ways to show respect for another person, please take some time to consider at least 4 more words that would describe respect for another person.

1)………………………………………………………………………………………………….

2)………………………………………………………………………………………………….

3)………………………………………………………………………………………………….

4)………………………………………………………………………………………………….

SLIDE SIX – Respect needs to be built into your everyday thinking and actions.

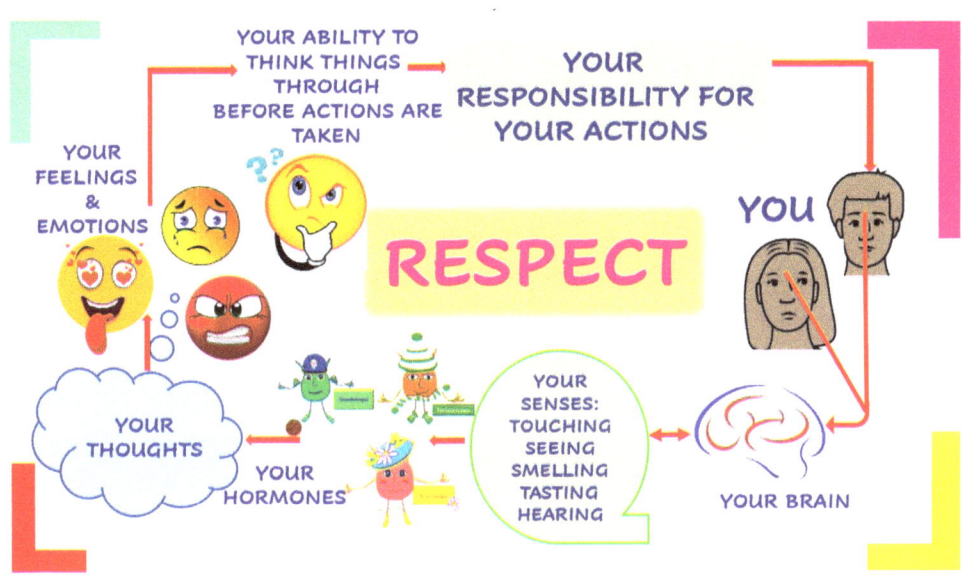

SLIDE SEVEN –
PEOPLE ARE DIFFERENT

We are one world community, we each look different through the colour of our skin, eyes, hair and have different characteristics, but we all function on the inside in similar ways. Each person has a heart, brain, lungs,

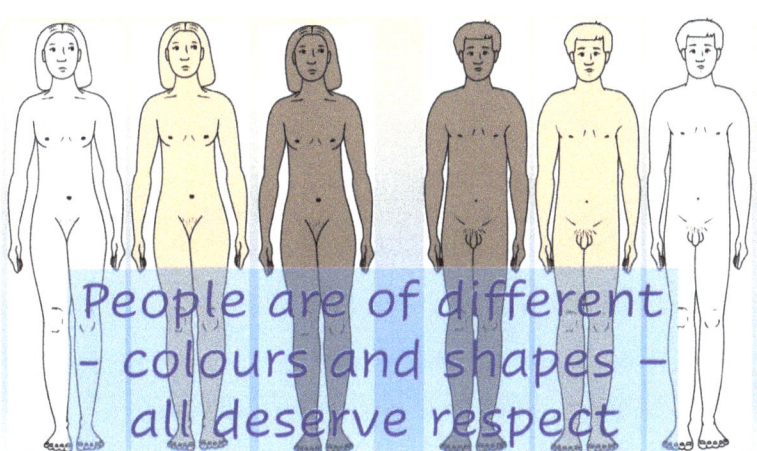

and other body parts that allow them to live their life and do the jobs they are meant to do. Some are born as biological females and some as biological males, some people are older and some younger, regardless of differences, each person deserves respect.

YOUR NOTES

....
....
....

SLIDE EIGHT – TAKING ON THOSE EMBARASSING WORDS…

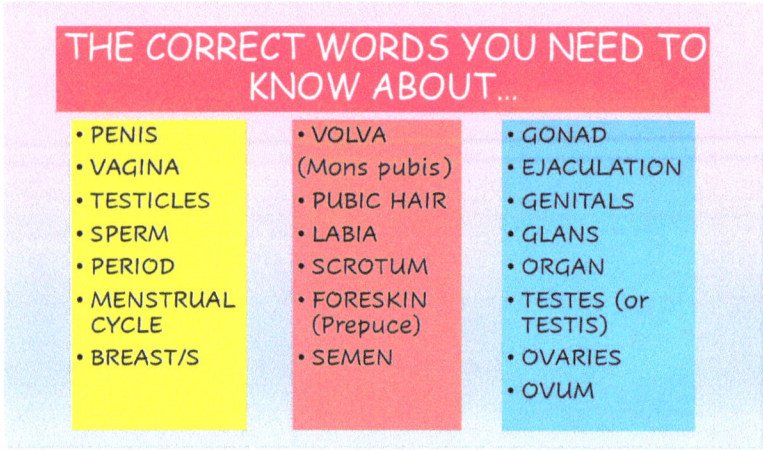

Many parts of the human body are given different names, and some are disrespectful. Whilst, at different times, this may be funny, it is important to remember, the body is a unique piece of human technology that has come together from your ancestors over many thousands of years and generations and this fact should not be forgotten. The main body's function is to keep you safe, and when the body comes under attack, the main function is to help you fight condition, as in Covid, or when breaking your bones, the function is to help your body heal. This is why, understanding the parts of your body that function in your health is important.

Each word is unique on the screen, so let's start: PENIS, VAGINA, TESTICLES, SPERM, PERIOD, MENSTRUAL CYCLE, BREAST/S, VOLVA, LABIA, SCROTUM, FORESKIN, SEMEN, GONAD, EJACULATION, GENITALS, GLANS, ORGAN, TESTES (OR TESTIS), OVARIES, OVUM.

Each word mentioned in these 3 lists has a purpose and function in your body.

YOUR NOTES

PENIS-each biological male born has a penis……………………………………

VAGINA-each biological female born has a vagina……………………………

TESTICLES-males have testicles………………………………………………………..

SPERM-males produce sperm in the testicles, sperm may make babies. It is the smallest cell in the human body………………………………………………

PERIOD-biological females have periods. A period is formed in the uterus, it is not life blood, but blood developed in the uterus for the purpose of making babies……………………………………………………………………….

MENSTRUAL CYCLE-is the process from the beginning to the end of each period cycle. Cycles can go from 21 to 35 days, depending on the female's body!…………………………………………………………………………………

BREASTS-both males and females have breasts. Females' breasts grow and develop differently because the purpose of breasts is to feed their babies with the milk the breast produce………………………………………………

VOLVA-is the mound that develops in the pubic area as the female grows and develops. The volva and pelvic bone area becomes stronger with puberty but is not as strong as a fully mature female. The pubic bone strength helps to protect the uterus and to carry an unborn child……………..

LABIA-is the soft flesh and is in folds which helps to protect the female's 2 body openings which are the urethra, where waste fluid is released, vagina, and anus. The anus in both males and females allows for the extraction of food waste from the body………………………………………………

SCROTUM-is the soft skin bags on a male that protect the testicles. The scrotum can expand during hot weather, this keeps the testes cool, and tighten in cold weather; this allows the testes to be kept warm………………

FORESKIN-the penis, when a baby boy is born, it completely covers the end of the penis. Depending on culture, religion, or choice, during a surgical operation, the foreskin is removed………………………………………………

SEMEN-is released from the prostate gland. Semen helps to protect the sperm; this whitish sticky substance allows the sperm to be recharged once they have left the testes and have travelled up the vas deferens. Semen is a combination of fructose, protein, and hormones. This highly charged combination of sticky liquid allows the sperm to continue its journey and reach its destination! It can be released involuntary, in and through 'wet dreams', which is a perfectly natural process for the male body to undertake and is a process that helps to keep the penis healthy. Releasing old sperm allows new sperm to be made………………………………………

GONAD/S- are sex glands in both male and females. The gonads' main function is to help to control the functions within the ovaries and testes.

EJECULATION-is the release of sperm from the penis. Release can take place through intercourse. Intercourse should only happen by two consenting, caring, and loving, adults at the appropriate ages. Keeping in mind, underage sexual activity is breaking the law and can end up with a prison sentence or being convicted of sexual crimes………………………………

GENITALS-both males and females have genitals. They are a private part of the human body and should always be respected………………………………….

GLANS & ORGAN-are other names for the penis.

TESTES OR TESTIS- are the testicles held in place by the male scrotum. Testes is the plural name for the two, and testis, the singular name for one! A male can still produce healthy, active sperm with one testis…………………

OVARIES-are where the female stores the eggs which may eventually help her to make her baby or babies. A female is born with her eggs. She is not like a male who continually makes or produces sperm………………………………

OVUM-is a mature female egg. It is the largest cell in the human body…..

YOUR NOTES – PLEASE RECAP ON THE INFORMATION
……
……

SLIDE NINE –THE DUAL SYSTEM OF CHILDHOOD INTO ADULTHOOD

During puberty and while your brain is still developing and changes are taking place to your body, at times you may feel a little bit lost. You want to take part in the adult conversations or actions, but in part of your thinking, you may want to go and play with your mates or friends! This is normal, even adults need to re-learn how to play! If, as a young person, you don't know what is happening to your brain, mind, and body, this may be the time a person gets into trouble with either their parents or the law…!

By keeping your brain, working, your mind active with positive projects such as sport, helping with the house chores, even helping with helping your parents in the garage, on the farm, in their business, or finding a part-time job, you will not become bored. Boredom gets young people into trouble within the community and the law!

This transition from teenager to adult is a necessary process into the adult world. Accordingly, *'A range of social determinants of health arise in adolescence, with peers, school, and eventually the workplace becoming strong determinants of health and well-being as the influence of the family wanes!'* (Viner and others 2012)

SLIDE TEN -TO RECAP – PLEASE TAKE NOTE.
IF YOU FEEL SOME OF THE FEELINGS OUTLINED IN THIS SLIDE, PLEASE TALK WITHIN THE GROUP OR WITH A MATURE AND RESPONSIBLE ADULT

DUAL SYSTEMS – TO RECAP:

THROUGH PUBERTY, AS WE GROW AND CHANGE, SOME OF THE OLD PARTS OUR PERSONALITY AND MEMORIES WANT TO GO BACK TO THE FUN TIMES OF CHILDHOOD, BUT SOME PARTS OF US KNOW WE HAVE A PART-TIME JOB AND KNOW:

'I HAVE TO GET READY TO GO TO WORK BECAUSE I WANT TO BUY THOSE TRAINERS, NETBALL EQUIPMENT OR YOU ARE SAVING UP TO BUY YOUR FIRST CAR...!'

THIS TYPE OF THINKING IS RELATED TO WAY YOUR BRAIN AND EMOTIONS ARE WORKING TOGETHER...

YOUR NOTES

....
....
....
....
....

SLIDE ELEVEN- THE MALE AND FEMALE BODY

The male and female biological bodies are different, and this difference is with good purpose and that purpose is to reproduce; some of you may, eventually, have a family and that then becomes an important part of your life; that is the reproduction cycle and of life.

THE FEMALE BODY – has three openings in the genital area of her body. The URETHRA, which allows her to release wastewater or pee/wee. The VAGINAL OPENING, which allows her to release the blood caused by a period and in the conception of making a child and having intercourse, and the ANAL area which allows her body to release the waste matter from eating solid food such as bread, vegetables, fruit, and other foods.

THE MALE BODY – has two openings in the genital area of his body. The URETHRA, which allows him to release the wastewater or pee/wee. The URETHRA also allows sperm to travel out of the penis when it is released. The ANAL area, which like the female, allows his body to release waste matter from eating solid food such as bread, vegetables, fruit, and other foods.

YOUR NOTES

....

....

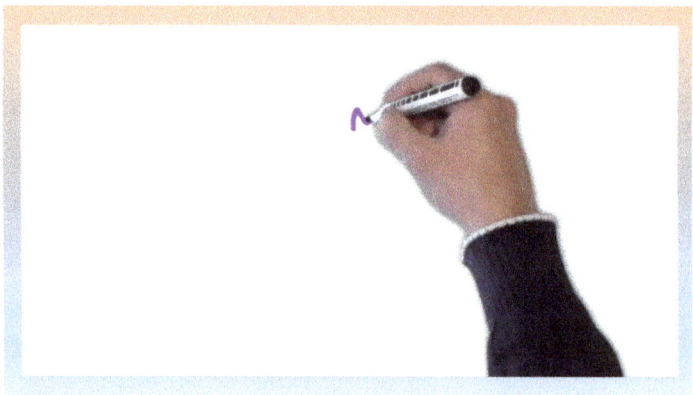

SLIDE TWELVE – WE ARE ALL DIFFERENT ON THE OUTSIDE, BUT SIMILAR ON THE INSIDE...

YOUR NOTES

....

....

....

....

THE FEMALE BODY

Prior to a female having her periods, her body and brain, like the male, has a lot of growing and maturing to do.

In both males and females, puberty is a process that goes on for several years. Your body and brain may start the process of puberty at six years of age. Because there are no visible signs that puberty is happening, the hormones inside your body may be on the move! Science and technology is now revealing more information about how the human body and brain grow and change through these formative years.

Please remember, you are receiving this information; this information needs to be treated with respect.

At puberty and throughout a female's reproductive years while her period takes place, there are Four Stages to each cycle:

SLIDE THIRTEEN- STAGE ONE - THE FEMALE MENSTRUATION CYCLE

This slide shows you how a female body grows. Here, you can see there is no blood forming in the uterus, this may be before a female starts her periods or at the start of a new cycle!

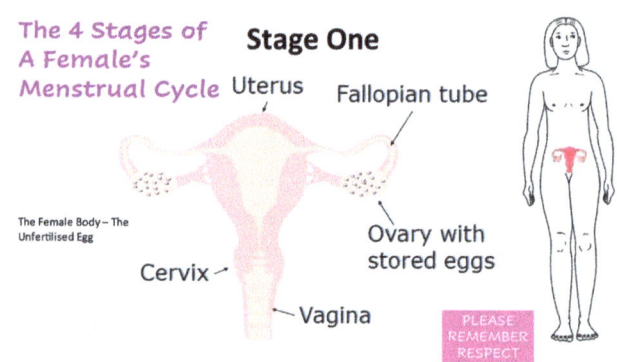

SLIDE FOURTEEN
- STAGE TWO – THE FEMALE MENSTRUATION CYCLE

In Stage Two, the lining of the wall of the uterus starts to thicken with a blood lining. The lining will continue to thicken as the female becomes closer to the period starting date. In this slide, you can see how the mature egg, (ovum), has left the ovary, and is travelling through the fallopian tube.

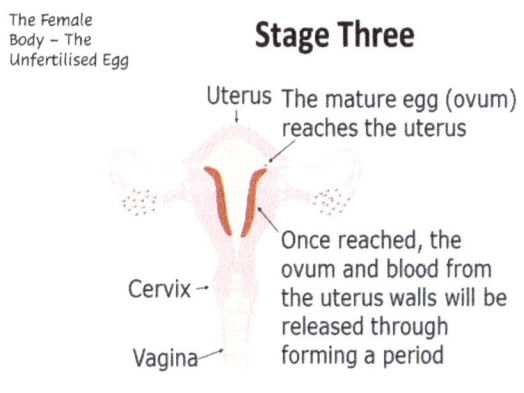

SLIDE FIFTEEN - STAGE THREE –THE FEMALE MENSTRUATION CYCLE

In Stage Three, the mature egg, (ovum) has reached the neck of the uterus and is about to enter the uterus which is a female reproductive organ. If the egg is not fertilised by a sperm, the egg will continue to travel into the uterus which action will release the blood covering the uterus wall.

SLIDE SIXTEEN– STAGE FOUR – THE FEMALE MENSTRUAL CYCLE

Stage Four, the blood is released from the walls of the uterus; this is the period.

The first period can be light in colour and only last a short time. Once the period has finished, the cycle begins again. There is no myth or intrigue to the female menstrual cycle. It is a normal function of the female body and should always the respected.

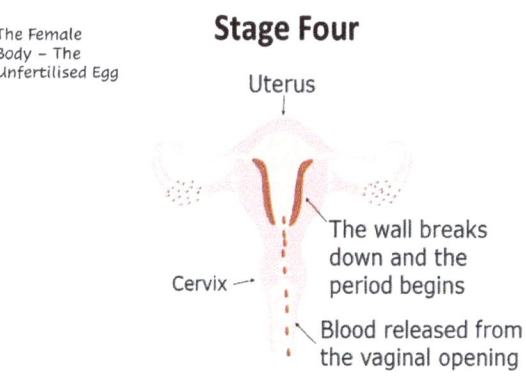

It takes hormones for the female body to work and stay healthy. Hormones are a natural part of life.

YOUR NOTES

....
....
....
....
....
....
....
....
....
....
....
....

SLIDE SEVENTEEN - THE COMPLETE FEMALE MENSTRUAL CYCLE
OPEN DISCUSSION IF APPROPRIATE

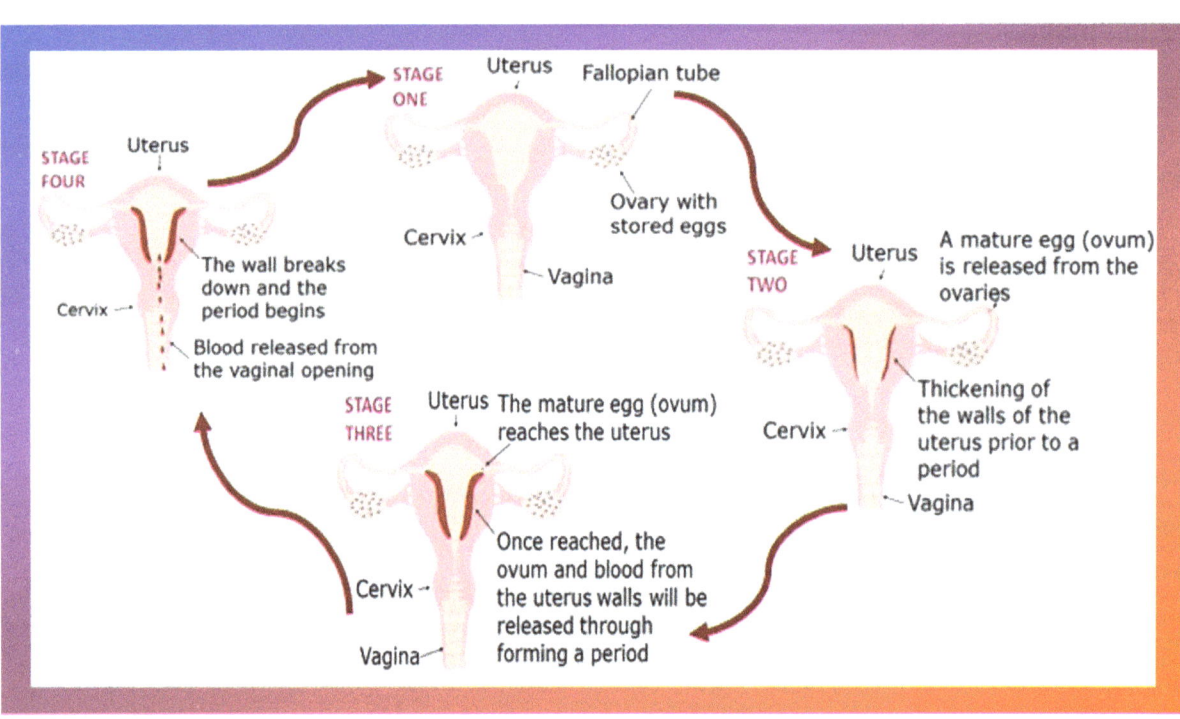

YOUR NOTES

....
....
....
....
....
....
....

Please Note
It was once thought, for a female to produce a baby, she needed to have a period, that is now proven to be incorrect. It is the release of the mature female egg into the fallopian tube, at that stage it has become the ovum, that allows conception to take place!

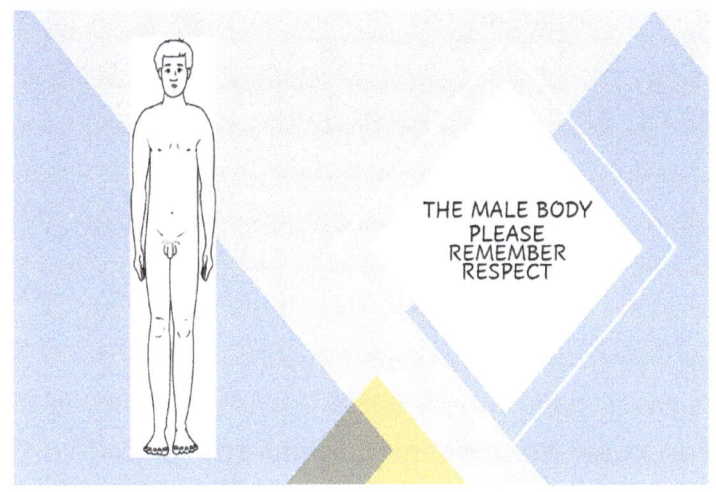

SLIDE EIGHTEEN – UNDERSTANDING HOW THE MALE BODY WORKS

All growth and puberty growth are driven by hormones. The role your hormones play can either keep you healthy or make you sick, this is true for both males and females. Like your body and brain, the hormones in your body need to be fed by healthy food.

YOUR NOTES

....
....
....

SLIDE NINETEEN – THE MALE BODY AND HOW IT WORKS…

1) The vas deferens, (number 7) is the tube that carries the sperm from the testes to the prostate gland.

2) The urethra is the tube that carries the urine; it is the waste from the fluids previously swallowed. On leaving the prostate gland, the sperm enters the urethra which allows it to travel and leave the penis.

3) is the penis and known as a glans, organ, or member.

4) is the bladder and is where urine is stored.

We each know when we need to go to the bathroom, because we each get a twinge or message to our brain saying, *'you need to go to the bathroom!'*

5) is the prostate gland and regulates the sperm when it travels up the vas deferens. By the time the sperm reaches the prostate gland, it becomes tired. The prostate supplies much needed energy for the sperm to carry on its journey.

6) is the scrotum, as a male enters puberty, the scrotum, like the penis, grows, it might also go darker in colour. The scrotum has the role to protect

the testes and sperm, therefore, it is loose in the summer heat but will tighten up when the body gets cold.

7) Testis. Two testis are called testes, and a singular is testis.

YOUR NOTES

....

....

....

SLIDE TWENTY - THE MALE PENIS

Like the female genital area, the male genitals also need to be shown respect.

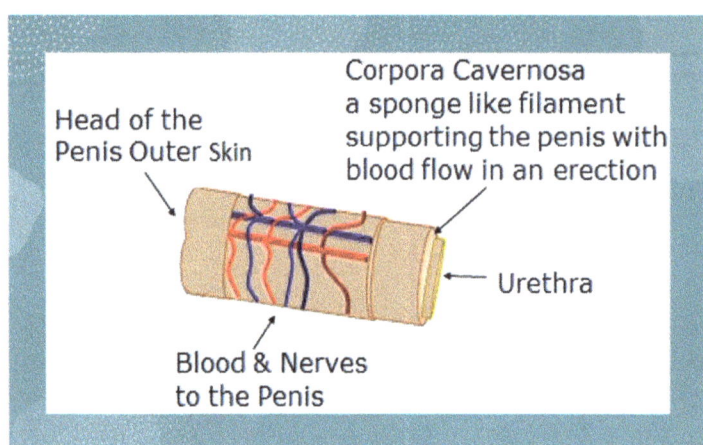

The male organ and genitals, like the female genitals is always a delicate area of the human body and, must be treated with respect.

For a male to gain an erection, the penis needs to fill with blood pumped from his body. An erection can be natural because the penis needs to release sperm; old sperm needs to be released at different times to allow new sperm to take its place!

The blood flow from the body fills the corpora cavernosa. This is a sponge like area, just like the sponge used for sucking up water in the sink; when filled with blood, this sponginess allows the penis to stiffen and become firm.

Both the penis and vagina are highly sensitive areas of the human body with your body's areas connected to your nervous system through the body's electronic network. The electronics from the genitals connect to the brain and this sends the messages which create the feelings, and sometimes the emotions, that allow two loving people to make love.

1) A male erection can be involuntary, which allows the body to release old sperm.
2) The Corpora Cavernosa is the sponge-like area in the penis that allows it to fill with blood.
3) Once the penis is erect, it can release sperm.
4) The penis, like the vagina, are highly sensitive to thought and touch.

SLIDE TWENTY-ONE - PLENARY

YOUR NOTES

....
....
....
....
....
....
....
....
....

PLENARY & REFLECTION ON THE INFORMATION YOU HAVE LEARNT

- The vital role that respect plays is in all aspects of life.
- How people of all different backgrounds, beliefs and different shapes deserve to be treated with respect at all times.
- How to appropriately use the correct terminology for different parts of the human body.
- The Dual systems of growth and maturity and how your brain is also growing and maturing as you go into and through puberty.
- How the menstrual cycle works within females and how their body starts to change as they progress into Womanhood
- The vital makeup and structure of the male penis.

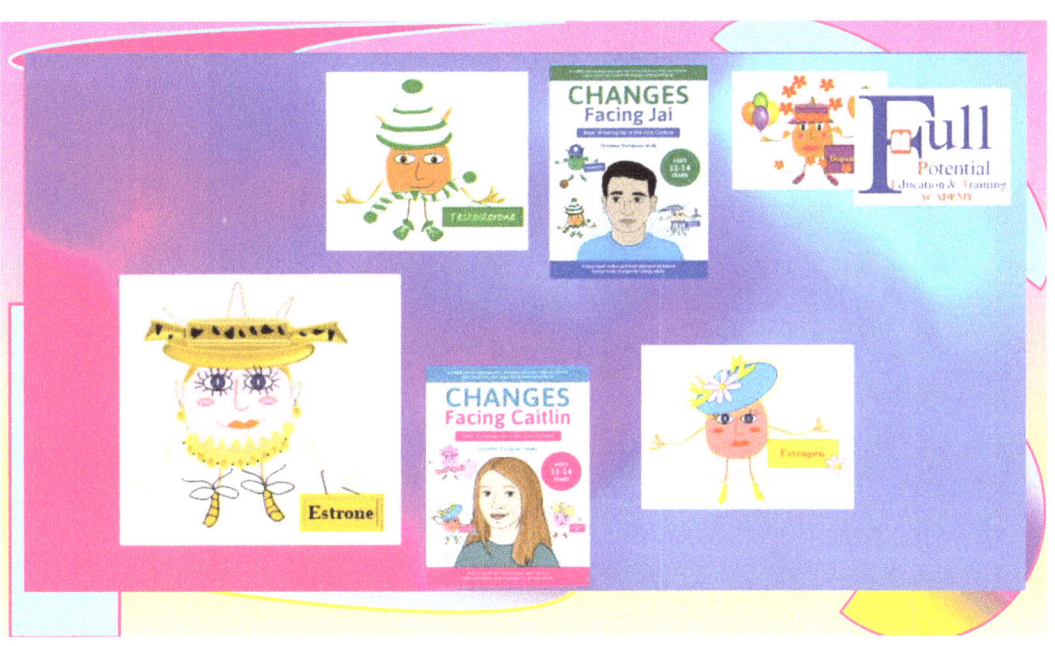

END OF SESSION TWO

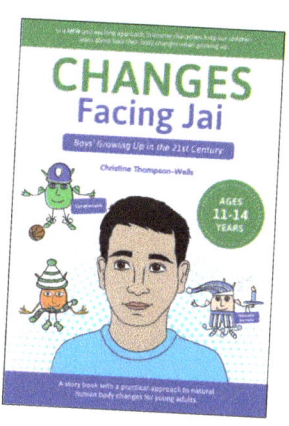 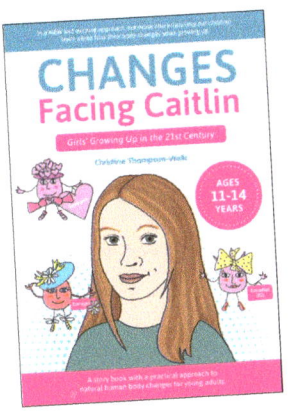

SEE YOU IN SESSION THREE

SESSION THREE
RESPECT, RESPONSIBILITIES & HORMONES
CHANGES TO THE HUMAN BODY AND BRAIN
THE JOURNEY OF PUBERTY

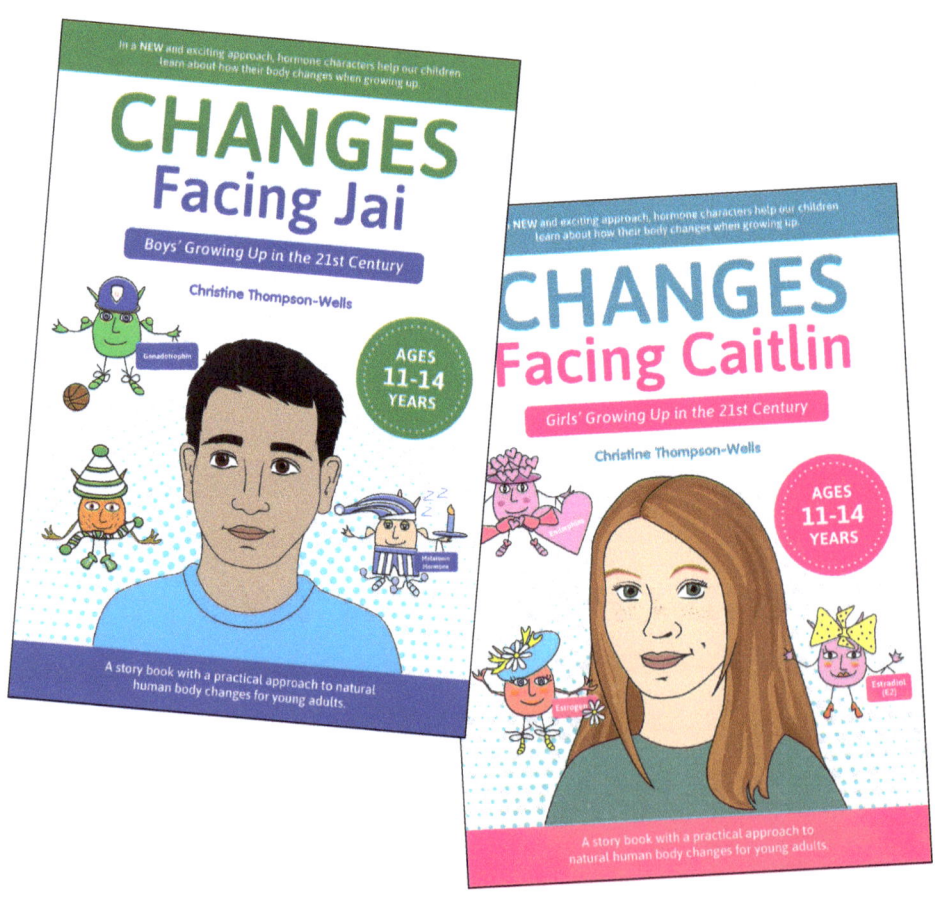

SLIDE ONE – THE JOURNEY OF PUBERTY WELCOME

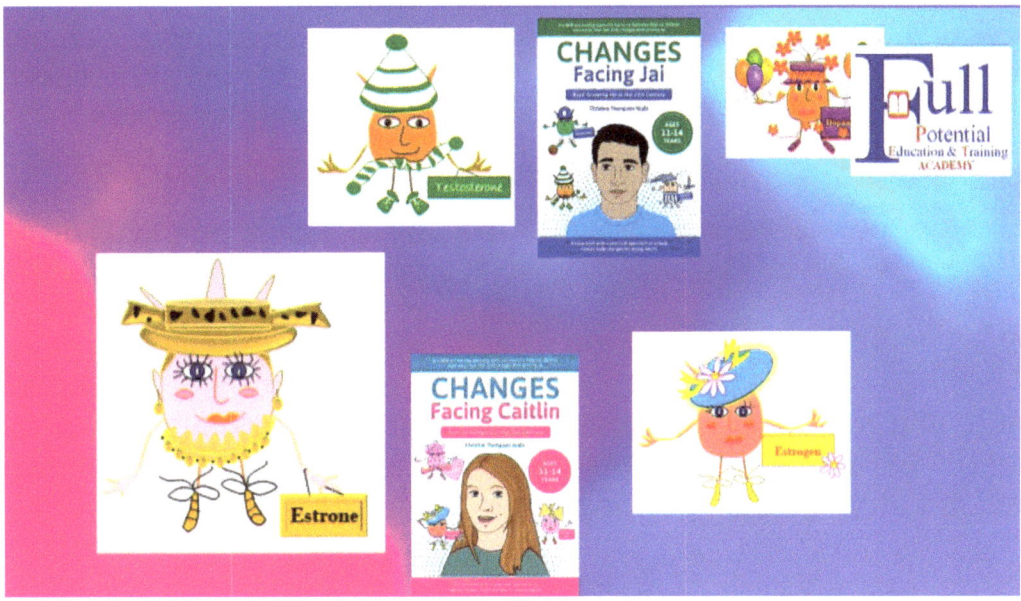

This session takes us into the 'How?' and 'Why?' of puberty and how the female and male develop differently within weeks after conception.

SLIDE TWO, HORMONES WITH HATS, SESSION THREE

It's strange to have hormones with hats but it is one way of identifying the hormone and for you to remember the work the hormone does within your body and brain!

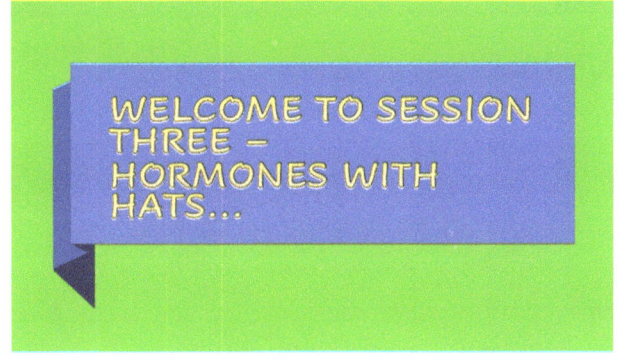

SLIDE THREE – INTRODUCTION VIDEO

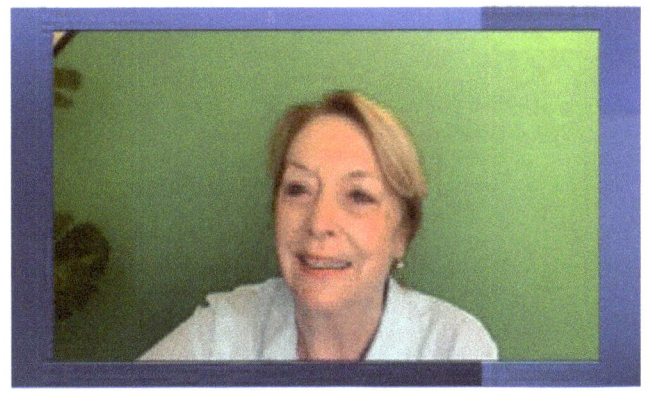

SLIDE FOUR – RESPECT

> **Respect**
> **OBJECTIVES AND OUTCOMES FOR THE SESSION**
>
> By the end of the session, you, the student, will have an understanding of how both the female and male bodies work when intercourse happens and the possible outcome of pregnancy.
>
> You will have a greater understanding of how the sex of a child happens and have knowledge and know the difference between the 'X' and 'Y' chromosomes. You will also understand the way that a child is conceived.
>
> By watching the birth of Isaacs, a real case study, you will gain a greater understanding of the responsibilities associated with adulthood and relationships.

Throughout the sessions, we have placed great emphasis on respect, that is respect for your body, for other people's bodies and for the role the human body plays in serving us through our lives and we cannot forget, the role of respect for our hard-working brains. Your brain loves to work but can only work properly if you treat it with respect. That is, always think about the habits you create. Be aware of eating junk food, taking drugs, consuming too much alcohol, trying vaping or any other habit that will interfere with your wellbeing.

SLIDE FIVE – THE CHANGING HUMAN MALE BODY

Every person has hormones working in their body. At this moment, at least one quarter of the world population is going through puberty, and is experiencing, similar experiences to you. Their body and brains are also changing….!

YOUR NOTES

....
....
....
....
....
....
....
....

People are of different colours, and shapes – Each deserves respect

SLIDE SIX – THE BIOLOGICAL MALE BODY IS DIFFERENT TO THE FEMALE BIOLOGICAL BODY…

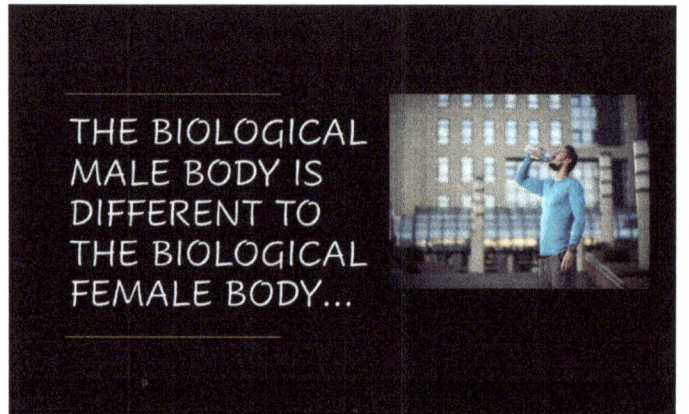

We each know that boys and girls, males and females are different! But how does that difference come about?

YOUR NOTES

....
....
....

SLIDE SEVEN THE DIFFERENCE BETWEEN MALES AND FEMALES

Biological males are different to biological females. All embryos start off as females and not males. It is the development, at about eight weeks into the pregnancy, which allows the 'Y' chromosome to develop. This development allows the hormone testosterone to form in the small male body.

Testosterone encourages the testes, and penis to grow and the brain to develop into the male brain.

As we know, males are different to females! Males have testicles and a penis and females have a vagina, uterus, and other female body parts, including breasts for feeding babies!

YOUR NOTES

....
....

SLIDE EIGHT – THE 'Y' CHROMOSOME MAKES THE DIFFERENCE – SO WHAT IS A CHROMOSOME?

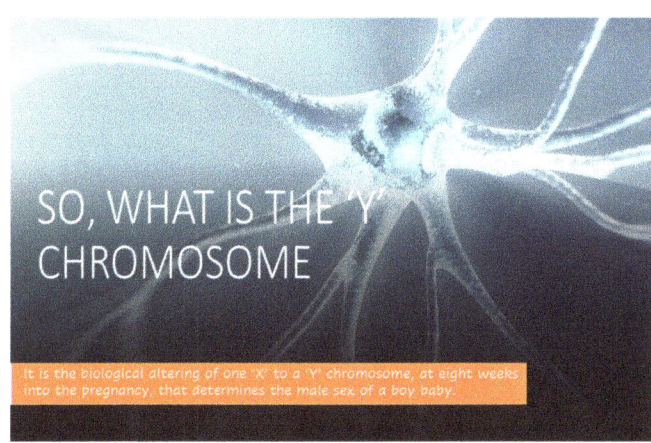

There are normally twenty-three pairs of chromosomes in each cell. While twenty-two pairs are called autosomes the twenty-third pair are known as the sex chromosomes. It is the biological altering of one 'X' to a 'Y' chromosome, at eight weeks into the pregnancy, that determines the male sex of a boy baby.

YOUR NOTES

....
....
....
....
....
....
....
....

SLIDE NINE – THE WORK OF THE CHROMOSOMES

Please take some time to study this slide and discuss with your class friends and family.

DISCUSSION

………………………….
………………………….
………………………….
………………………….

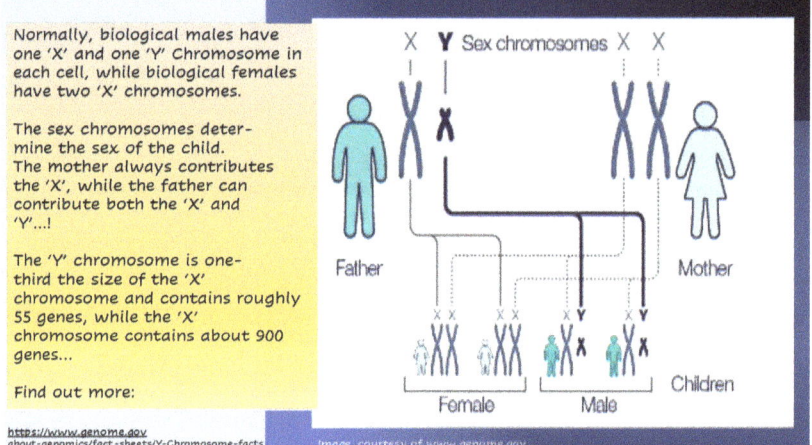

SLIDE TEN – THE FEMALE BODY IS DIFFERENT TO THE MALE BODY

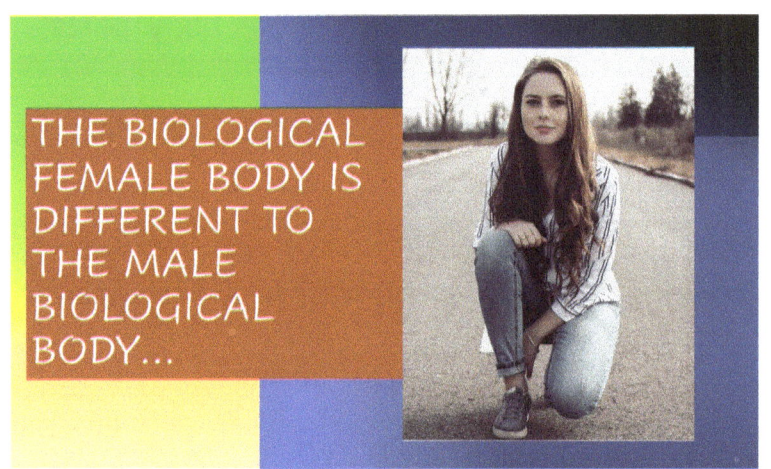

The difference between both males and females is for good reason, it is to allow the human species to survive!

YOUR NOTES

………………………………..
………………………………..
………………………………..
………………………………..
………………………………..

SLIDE ELEVEN – MALE AND FEMALE BODY'S ARE DIFFERENT

Male sex organs are on the outside of the body, and female sex organs are mainly on the inside of the body, this is the main difference in the species.

On the outside of the female body, we see the breasts or mammary glands. These glands are intended, by nature, to feed a baby.

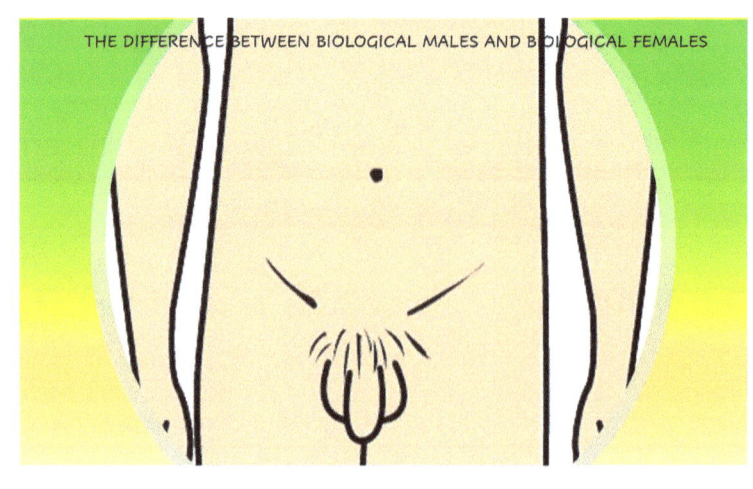

YOUR NOTES

………………………………………………………………………………………

SLIDE TWELVE – STAGE ONE – THE DIFFERENCE – THE FEMALE BODY AND REPRODUCTION – MATURE EGG ENTERS THE FALLOPIAN TUBE

At the beginning of the journey, the mature egg (ovum) starts to travel through the fallopian tube.

YOUR NOTES

………………………………….
…………………………………..
…………………………………..
…………………………………..
…………………………………..
…………………………………..
…………………………………..

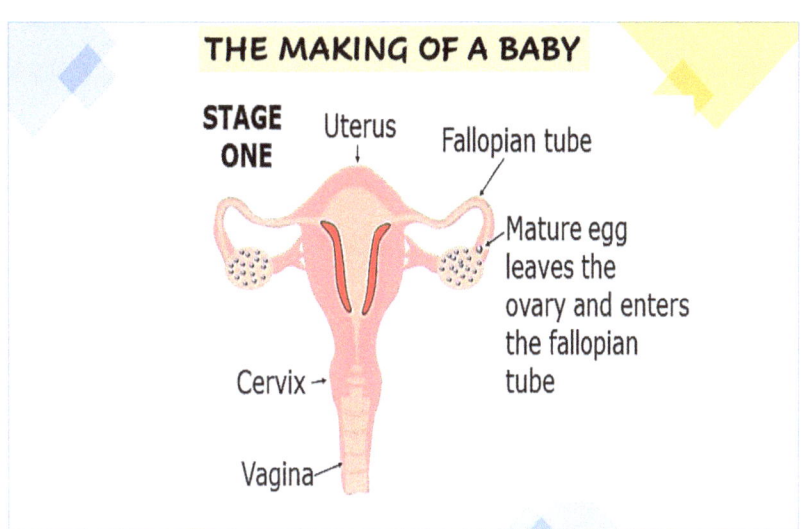

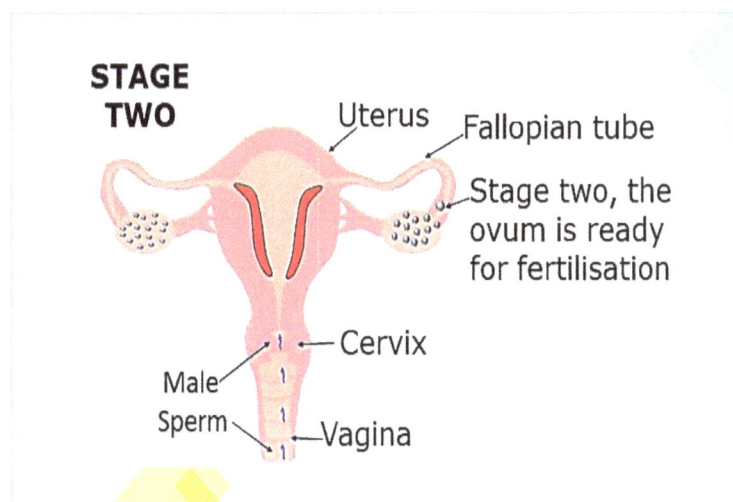

SLIDE THIRTEEN – STAGE TWO

After intercourse, the sperm travels up the female vagina to meet the mature egg, (ovum). If the ovum meets the sperm in the fallopian tube, and a connection is made, pregnancy may be the outcome.

SLIDE FOURTEEN – STAGE THREE

During intercourse, a healthy male may release between 40 million to 1.2 billion sperm cells. It takes one sperm to fertilize the female egg/ovum.

DISCUSSION

………………………………
………………………………

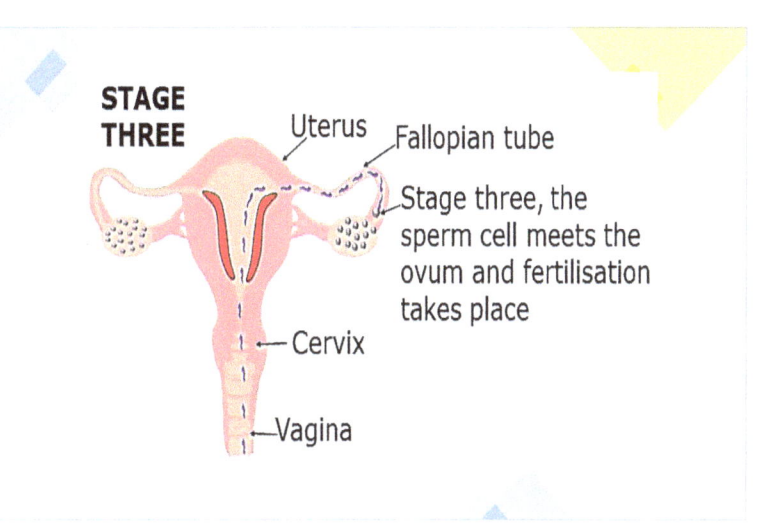

SLIDE FIFTEEN – THE FOUR PHASES OF THE SPERM JOURNEY

In this phase, the strongest sperm reaches the egg and is ready to fertilise the ovum. The outer rim of the female egg has a mucus edging, this helps to protect and keep the egg safe as it goes on the journey within the female body.

YOUR NOTES

……………………………………….
……………………………………….
……………………………………….
……………………………………….
……………………………………….

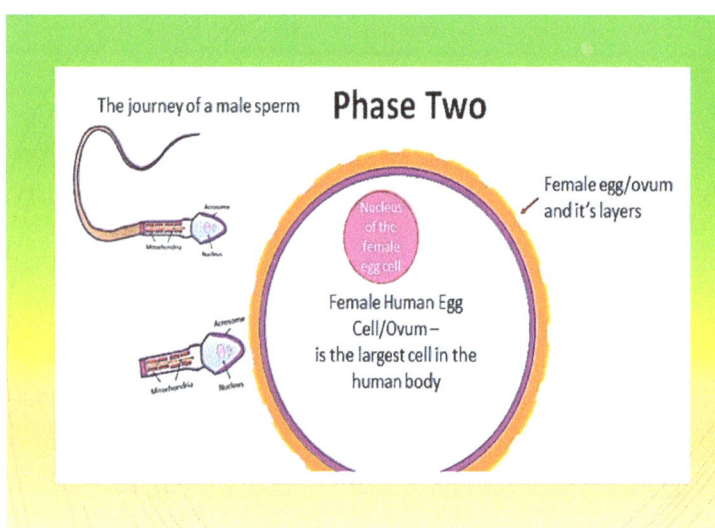

SLIDE SIXTEEN – PHASE TWO

Within the second phase, the sperm loses its tail and the head of the sperm, which has an enzyme edge; (this can be seen in purple on the slide). The enzyme allows the head to burrow through the mucus and outer rim of the female ovum, this allows fertilization to take place.

SLIDE SEVENTEEN – PHASE THREE

Within the head of the sperm lies the nucleus. The female ovum has its own nucleus; once both nuclei meet, this then becomes a power engine that work as one.

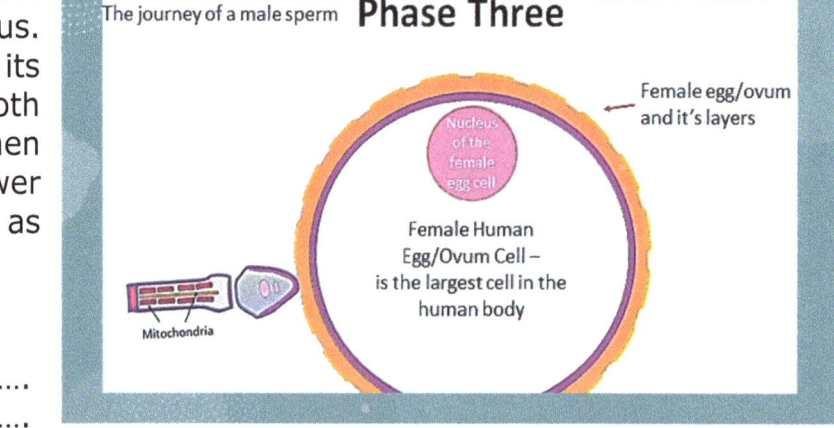

YOUR NOTES

……………………………………….
……………………………………….
………………………………………………………………………………………….

SLIDE EIGHTEEN – PHASE FOUR

Both nuclei have connected and now the coming together to continue to divide and multiply. Once the multiplying of cells in the fallopian tube has taken place, the bundle is ready to move down to the uterus!

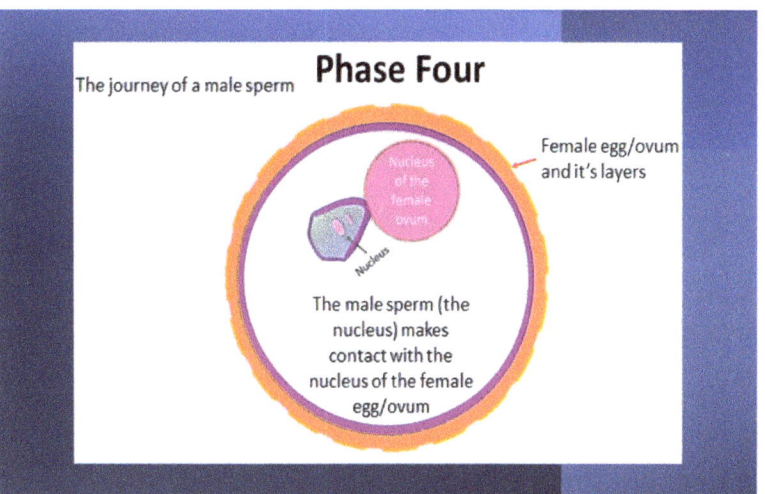

SLIDE NINETEEN – ACTIVATION AND CONNECTION OF TWO HUMAN CELLS

In Diagram One, and at the start of fertilization, the male sperm and female ovum have connected. As seen in the previously spoken about phases; the sperm has penetrated the outer rim of the ovum, allowing the pregnancy to proceed. Once the two cells, (the sperm and ovum) are as one, the one cell divides into two.

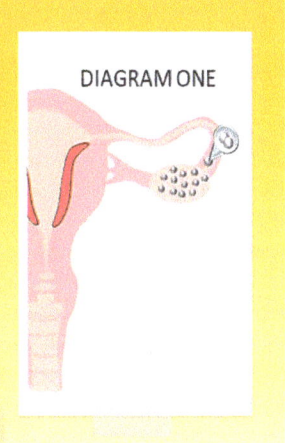

In this slide, the male sperm and female ovum have connected. As seen in the previously spoken about phases, the sperm has penetrated the outer rim of the ovum, allowing the pregnancy to proceed.

YOUR NOTES

……………………………………..
……………………………………..
……………………………………..
………………………………………………………………………………………..

SLIDE TWENTY – THE CELLS CONTINUE TO DIVIDE AND MULTIPLY WHILE IN THE FALLOPIAN TUBE

In the early stages, the bundle may resemble the appearance of a raspberry. In diagram two, the division of cells continues.

YOUR NOTES

……………………………………..
……………………………………..
……………………………………..
……………………………………..
………………………………………………………………………………………..
………………………………………………………………………………………..

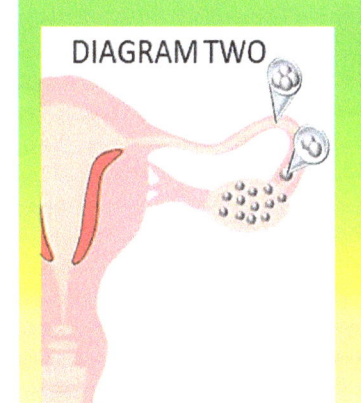

In the early stages, the bundle may resemble the appearance of a raspberry.
In diagram two, the division of cells continues.

SLIDE TWENTY-ONE – REINFORCING THE JOURNEY

In diagram three, the cells continue to divide and multiply.

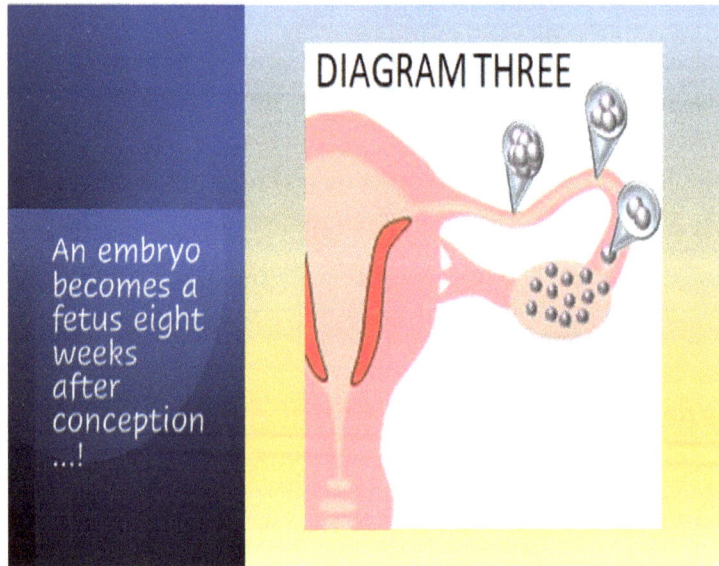

For the healthy development of the bundle, the mother needs to feel secure, have the correct amount of rest, eat a healthy, sustainable diet of fresh food containing the correct fats, complex carbohydrates, unadulterated fats (natural fats), and healthy quantities of water.

SLIDE TWENTY-TWO –
THE CELL BUNDLE ATTACHES TO THE UTERUS WALL

Once the connection is made to the uterus, the mother's blood supply will feed into the bundle allowing the pregnancy to continue.

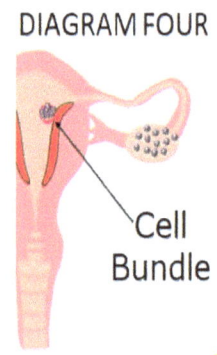

In Diagram four, the bundle travels down the fallopian tube and connects to the wall of the female uterus.

A pregnancy usually lasts 40 weeks but some babies come early and some a little later...

YOUR NOTES

....

....

....

SLIDE TWENTY-THREE – THE GROWTH AND PROGRESSION OF AN EMBRYO

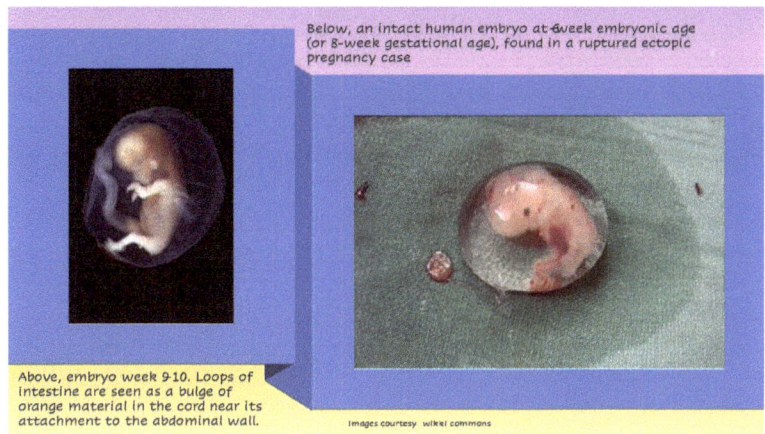

At all times, the respect for the sexual act should be observed. People who naturally love each other will want to make love, but if sex is performed without respect, the development of a human life may be the outcome.

SLIDE TWENTY-FOUR – THE BIRTH OF ISAAC – 14 MINUTE VIDEO

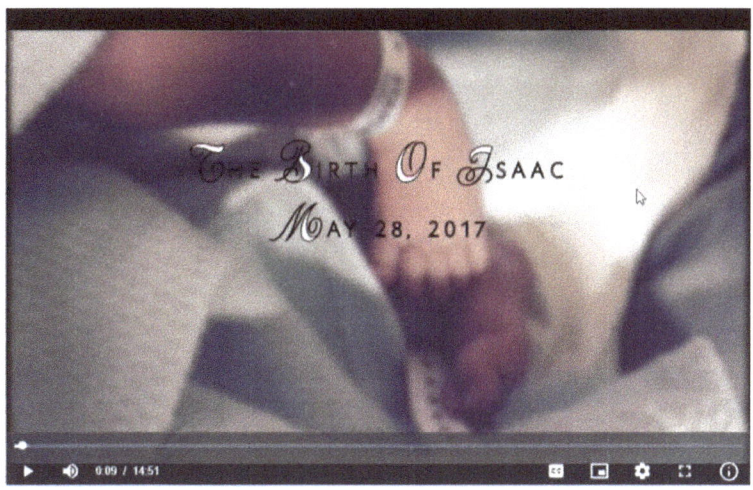

Acknowledgement and thank you to Wiki Commons and Isaac's mum for producing this beautiful video.

DISUSSION

YOUR NOTES

……………………………………
……………………………………
……………………………………
……………………………………

TWENTY-FIVE – PLENARY

YOUR NOTES

……………………………………
……………………………………
……………………………………
……………………………………
……………………………………
……………………………………
……………………………………
……………………………………
……………………………………

PLENARY & REFLECTION ON THE INFORMATION YOU HAVE LEARNT

We have discussed many aspects of puberty during our 3 Sessions together, let's now reflect on this last Session

✓ Respect has been at the forefront of the information spoken about during our 3 Sessions together
✓ We have discussed chromosomes
✓ How human fertilisation takes place
✓ The progression the human sex cells make form an embryo
✓ Development of the embryo, and the
✓ Birth of Isaac
✓ Summing Up

SLIDE TWENTY-SIX – CONCLUSION OF SESSIONS

YOUR NOTES

....
....
....
....
....
....
....
....
....
....
....
....
....
....

ALWAYS TAKE A MOMENT….

Always take a moment to think before you act; think about the consequences of your actions. Outcomes of unthought about actions and sexual activities may be the transfer of Sexually Transmitted Diseases, (STD'S), unwanted pregnancies, hurt and pain of another person.

Underage sexual activities are a criminal act; there are severe outcomes for breaking the law. If you have respect in your mind, you will not get into trouble.

Thank you for your attendance and for enjoying the journey of puberty. Stay safe, keep well and please remember, your brain is an obedient servant, it will always do what you command it to do, therefore, only give it good, positive commands and direction.

BUILDING LIFESKILLS IS A WAY OF KEEPING YOU SAFE.

CHRISTINE

Our Mission:
Every child and adult have value and is important to us; therefore, we strive through research, online education, and book publishing, to bring life-skill education to all children and all families.

For Education Packages

Please see our book website:
www.how2books.com.au and
Education packages,
www.fullpotentialtraining.com.au
or Contact:
admin@fullpotentialtraining.com.au

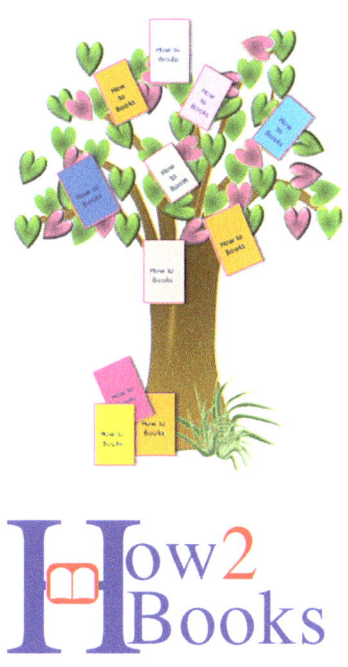

Education to keep our children and young adults safe...

www.ingramcontent.com/pod-product-compliance
Lightning Source LLC
Chambersburg PA
CBHW061537010526
44107CB00066B/2891